How to Manage Stress

The Six-Pillar Guide to Living Life With More Energy And Less Stress

Scott Michael Beech

Copyright

This book is not intended to replace, nor offer, any medical advice. This includes the diagnosis and treatment of illness.

Copyright © 2020 by Scott Michael Beech
Published and Printed Through Kindle Direct Publishing
First Edition, 2020

ISBN: 9798565449921

To order, visit Amazon Website

Thank You

I dedicate this book to my Dad, Mark,
who when I was younger, said,
"managing stress is everything." Then
when he saw that I was writing this
book, he said, "That's gonna be one of
the best books ever written."

Thanks Pop!

Table of Contents

Part 1 ~ The Power of Stress

Part 2 ~ On Balance

Part 3 ~ The Six Pillars...

Part 4 ~ How to Manage Stress

Foreward

There are several staples of healthy living, which, if a person can become skilled at, will contribute to a rich, healthy, and fulfilling life. Managing stress is one of these.

The other staples of healthy living include, but are not limited to: proper diet, exercise, social support, spiritual well-being, meaningful work, sleep, and taking care of the mind.

Out of all of these, diet and exercise are really the first two that have 'caught fire' in the United States. When I go into my local Barnes & Noble bookstore, I have noticed that there are dozens and dozens of books written on the subjects of diet and exercise for sale. It's not so easy to find books on the topic of managing stress.

The reason that the subjects of diet and exercise are so popular is because these two areas of health play a major role in how a person looks externally. If you have lived in the United States for any length of time, you have likely realized that external appearances have become near obsessions.

While there is nothing wrong with looking good and it's awesome for people to take care of their bodies; I also hope to see American's become just as obsessed with how they feel on the inside, as how they look on the outside. In order to feel good on the inside, taking care of the mind, expressing the emotions constructively, and *managing stress* will all be paramount.

My knowledge of stress management, which was needed for the writing of this book, basically comes from three places. The first is form my own experience of being burnt-out from too much stress The second is from reading hundreds of materials on the topic of stress including: articles, research papers, and books. And the third is from my experience talking about stress with people as a Certified Health Coach.

Foreward

During my earlier years of life, feeling overworked and stressed-out were companions that kept revisiting me. This is likely owed to the fact that I have a very 'Type A' personality, struggle with 'the condition' of perfectionism, and have gone through some heartbreaking experiences related to grief.

It's been said that people with a chronic illness become more expert on their condition than the doctors that they visit for treatment. In my case, chronic stress became almost like an illness, and I wanted to learn as much as I could on the subject matter, so that I could 'beat' my illness. After learning a lot about this "illness" I wanted to help others beat it, so that they could feel healthy and at peace, as I have more recently.

I have a business where I help people to talk about, and better manage, their stress levels. I wanted to provide my clients with some reading materials on the topic, such as a book, but I didn't love what was available. Some of the books I found on stress management were too heavily laden with scientific data and weren't very practical for day-to-day living. Others, I felt, were a little too heavily focused on diet and nutrition and didn't give enough importance on putting the body into the *relaxation response*. A few books on stress management were just 'out there.'

So I wrote my own book to provide to my clients. My intention here is to explain complex physical processes very simply, give insight into what happens to the body under stress, and to provide a lot of good strategies and insights to help others manage their stress levels. You too can use the information shared in this book to your advantage.

Part 1 of this book is titled *The Power of Stress* and will explain how and why stress occurs, explain the body's three modes of functioning in regards to stress, and describe the longer-term effects of chronic stress.

Part 2 will 'lighten things up' by explaining how to come into balance, the amazing effects that triggering relaxation can have on a person's body and mind, and will talk a little on the relationship between personality types and stress.

Part 3 is by far the largest section of the book, because I wanted to talk about how to manage stress much more than how it is caused and what it does. I wanted to keep the information in this book as optimistic and as hopeful as possible. The *six pillars of stress management* described in Part 3 are all helpful things that myself and others have done to live with more energy and less stress.

Part 4 of this book really ties everything together and allows a person to coach themselves from stressful-living to more enjoyable living.

While *How to Manage Stress* has a certain flow of information if read from cover-to-cover, it's not necessarily important to do so. Feel free to skip around in the book, and especially to jump right into Part 3 with the *six pillars* if you would like to do so. Then, if there are certain headings that really grab your attention, you can come back to those later.

At times, discussing the topic of chronic stress and the negative consequences that it can have on the body and mind can feel a bit 'heavy.' These topics are thoroughly discussed in Part 1, and if you do feel like they are causing you either sadness or anxiety, feel free to skip ahead in the book. This information is simply provided so that if a person *is* suffering the ill-effects of runaway distress, they can gain valuable insights and make key connections. Part 2 of this book, and onward, are much more optimistic and provide as much hope and encouragement as possible, for anyone who knows that they need to better manage their stress levels.

Bolded words will have definitions in the Glossary that can be found after Part 4 (page 203).

Introduction

I know what it's like to feel stressed-out; like REALLY stressed out. Chronic stress affects each of us a little differently, but for me, it leaves me feeling as though I have no energy, even if I can get a full night of sleep. It also causes my immune system to be diminished, I have difficulty enjoying the simple pleasures in life, and the world around me becomes pale.

I know what it's like to feel really stressed out, but I also know what it's like to recover from being stressed out. I know what it's like to take the winding road back to recovering your lost energy, and how, along the way, you can also recover your enjoyment of life, sense of beauty, and peace of mind.

Stress can be a term that's difficult to define, but generally speaking, a *stressful event* is one that triggers the activation of the fight or flight response in the nervous system. This response causes the heart to race, breathing to be shallow, and the higher reasoning centers of the brain to shut down. A small or moderate amount of stress can be a healthy thing for people to experience, as it gears us up for action and helps us to feel invigorated. Problems arise when the fight or flight response is activated for too long or too often. This can lead to feelings of distress and exhaustion due to chronic stress and fatigue.

In this day and age, it's become all too common for individuals to either feel chronically stressed or burnt out. According to an article from the *Journal of Applied Social Psychology*, men's level of perceived stress has risen by 29 percent from 1983 to 2009, while women's level of perceived stress has risen by 18 percent in the same time period. It appears that our technological advances have made life simpler in many ways, but have also pushed individuals farther apart and caused life to move at an unadaptable pace for many.

Young adults are the age group reporting the highest levels of stress, and even children as young as 8 are reporting unhealthy stress levels. We are nearing a time in our society where we must come to terms with our unhealthy level of stress and make a change. These changes start on the individual level as more people begin to say, "enough is enough!" to unhealthy stress levels. People will find that it's perfectly possible to live a rewarding life- full of work, family, and friends- and to feel happy rather than stressed. This book will teach you how.

Stress in America - A Snapshot

I have been doing extensive research on the topic of stress over the last several years. As part of this, I have also been studying the stress levels of people living in the United States. Since 1983 The APA (American Psychological Association) has been routinely surveying Americans to discover our major sources of stress and also how high we as Americans perceive our stress levels to be. Here is a summary of these findings:

- Stress levels have steadily risen since 1983 for all age groups except for people aged 65 and older. This likely indicates that as people age they develop coping mechanisms to better handle stressful events.
- Women's stress levels are higher than those of men.
- Minorities' stress levels are slightly higher than those of Caucasians.
- Young adults (18 to 33) have the highest stress levels of any age group followed by teens, and stress tends to go down as adults age.
- Unemployed people experience more stress than employed people, and older retired people have less stress than the employed.
- The adage that money can't buy happiness is still true, but greater income does tend to decrease stress levels. The

stress-reducing effects of greater income tend to level off around the $75,000 per household/per year mark.

Sources of Stress

Money and financial concerns tend to be the greatest source of stress for Americans every year. Approximately 70% of Americans report some level of stress surrounding money each year.

The second highest source of stress is usually work related and pertains to feeling overwhelmed at work, having too much to do, and having difficulty getting along with coworkers/managers.

Housing costs are a major source of stress for young adults, and older adults (65+) generally rate health concerns as their major source of stress. Teens don't feel as stressed about their health as older adults, but they do rate getting along with friends and finding a good college as major sources of stress.

Teens, more so than ever, are also rating climate change and the future of our nation as major sources of stress in their lives.

A big source of either joy or stress comes from our relationship with others. Each year approximately 55% of Americans say that family and/or romantic relationships are causing them stress. Loss of romantic relationships and divorce can be very stressful events in a person's life.

As I am writing this book, it is 2020 and stress from the Covid-19 pandemic is also being felt by many people across the world.

A Personal Journey

We all have daily sources of stress to deal with, and some days this stress may feel overwhelming. At other times we may go through periods of intense stress that can be triggered by the loss of a job, an accident, an unexpected medical diagnosis, the loss of a loved one, or even the death of a trusted pet. These events can cause major upheaval in our lives, and cause us to fall apart on the inside, before we hopefully rise back up again.

I have gone through three periods of intense stress in my life. The first began for me at just twelve years of age. There I was, a gangly twelve year old beginning my transition from boyhood to manhood commonly known as puberty. During puberty, a person's body parts tend to fit together kind of awkwardly, some facial features are disproportionate in size compared to the others, and the hormones begin a major shift in different directions.

Puberty is a time when the physical demands on the body to grow and transform also cause us to feel more sensitive to stress, as most of our resources are being deployed to help us grow.

For me, I felt very mentally and emotionally uncomfortable with transitioning from boyhood to manhood. This transition was so uncomfortable, that it became a big source of concern for me. I also started to look at members of the opposite sex differently than before. I even had a major crush on one of the girls in my class.

My fear of telling this girl how I felt about her, coupled with all the other concerns that I had about transitioning out of childhood, ended up being very stressful for me. I started having difficulty falling asleep at night, I had an ulcer arise in my stomach, and I just generally felt tired and low on energy. These physical symptoms were no doubt caused by a combination of physical stress from puberty plus the mental and emotional stress that I was feeling inside.

My mother, being concerned about my physical symptoms, brought me to the only place that people generally go with health concerns- the hospital. Unfortunately, the doctors there didn't really understand what was wrong with me and had little idea of how to help me. They didn't ask me about my thoughts and feelings, and since they didn't ask, I didn't tell.

Modern hospitals and clinics tend to be amazing places to go in cases of emergency, or when a life-saving surgery needs to be administered. Unfortunately, they are often very poor places to go if too much stress is the cause of your discomforts. Doctors do not normally have the time, or desire, to speak with people about their stress levels, even though stress is a major cause of 60 to 80 percent of hospital visits. In hospitals, the connection between mind and body is given little respect.

It's also very common that when physical discomforts are caused by stress, people do not make this connection. At twelve years old I considered my difficulty sleeping and ulcer in my stomach to simply be caused by 'bad luck'.

As time went on, I fortunately began to feel a sense of comfort with my transition through puberty. I even ended up telling that girl I liked how I felt. It was fortunate for me that she also liked me back, but I think that no matter the result of my confession, it was reliving to get my feelings 'off of my chest.'

The next period of overwhelming stress I went through is one very common with people in this day and age- feeling stressed out from doing too much and being too busy.

At the time, it was my second year of college, I was 20 years old, and I felt that I was doing everything I needed to do to be living a fulfilling life. As a result, I ended up doing too much of everything. I was an excellent student working hard with my 16 credits and getting all A's, I was seeing my friends almost every day, I had a girlfriend that I liked and who expected a lot of my time and attention, and I was generally exercising every single day, and partying every weekend. To fit all of these demands into my busy day I would always stay up until 1 a.m. or later. After not enough sleep, I would then wake up at 7 am or 8 am to fill up another day.

Now, none of these things I mentioned previously are in themselves bad things. It's great to have relationships, and it's awesome to be surrounded by friends. It's good to have meaningful work and to pursue the dream of getting a degree. Physical exercise can be good for the body, mind, and emotions.

But I was doing too much of all these things, and I didn't understand the concept of balance. A truly fulfilling life will include a balance of deep rest and activity. The body/mind/spirit of an individual will eventually grow weary if a person is constantly doing things, and not giving their systems time to recover.

Balance and rest weren't principles of enjoyable living that I understood at this time, and because of this, I ended up over-extending myself. Eventually, I was really exhausted. I had hit the point of physiological stress known as 'burnout'. After a semester of this furious pace, I went home to rest for three weeks over Christmas break. Now, three weeks of rest may sound restorative, but even after those three weeks, I still felt nearly wiped-out. I had worn myself out with stress.

My exhaustion and lack of energy eventually caused my romantic relationship to end, as I was constantly moody and had very little to offer. The stress from this break-up added to the stress that I was already feeling. Severe stress can really weaken the immune system and I started to experience frequent colds and sinus infections.

I was tired, sick, and in the dumps… A line from a popular music artist resonated with me that said, "I'm just so sick and tired of being sick and tired."

Eventually, I decided that something had to change. I couldn't get much enjoyment out of living this fast-paced, 'fulfilling life' anymore, so I began experimenting with ways that I could improve my condition.

One of the things that really helped me out was keeping a record of how well I felt each day so that I could get an idea of what I was doing on the days where I felt "healthy and well."

I realized that I was feeling better on days where I had a good balance between work, sleep, and friends; not just all work, friends, and more work. This realization caused me to really sit down and contemplate what was important to me, and, what I could cut back on.

What I ended up deciding, was that going to class and getting good grades was really important to me, so I continued this habit. I also still spent time with friends and family, but not as much. I still exercised, but not as often, or as intensely. I still dated… but not as frequently. I hollowed out time in my schedule to just sit around and read for enjoyment. I kept cutting back on things that I could live without so that I could get a full eight hours of sleep every night.

And I recovered.

The energy that I had lost, eventually came back. I started to really enjoy the present moment rather than constantly chasing something that was perennially out of reach. My life, and my health, drastically improved.

This was a good period in my life with a balance between time spent with friends and family, time alone, time studying, and time dating. I still felt successful, and for me, my grades proved that, but I also had more energy and I wasn't exhausted.

This was a good period in my life, but it didn't last for long. Everything that I was doing was really helping me, but then tragedy hit. In April of 2012, my younger sister committed suicide.

I was definitely not ready to say goodbye to this person, nor was I prepared for the trauma of losing someone that I loved in such a dramatic fashion. This kick-started the third major period of stress in my life, and the effects of this traumatic experience were felt strongly for a few years afterward.

After my sister passed, I somehow finished the semester of college that I was in; but it was very challenging. I then attempted to go to college the following semester, but I ended up dropping out. I dropped out for two reasons: the grief of losing someone that I loved made focusing on my studies very difficult, but I also started to notice something…

I noticed that a lot of my professors and classmates seemed to be living their lives with a moderate to a high amount of stress like I had been. They often seemed like they didn't have a lot of *zest* for life. Maybe you feel this way currently (like you've lost your *zest*), or you've noticed that this is the way life appears to be for most people. Either way, I knew that what I really wanted was to live life more fully. In a lot of ways, my inner spark and my desire to live life more fully were actually awakened by my sister's passing. So I dropped out of college.

After dropping out of school I moved back home with my family so that we could grieve and recover together. I also began asking myself the big questions about what I wanted from life.

From the outside, it looked like I wasn't doing too well. I dropped out of school, I was separated from my friends, and I was living in the middle of nowhere on a farm.

Although things didn't look very promising from the outside, I was actually handling things pretty well given the circumstances. The commitments that I had made to better managing my stress levels in the year prior really acted as a buffer to the loss I was experiencing. Not only did I continue to make time for myself and schedule my days effectively; I also raised my commitments to my stress management practices. I began meditating every single day, and eight years later, I continue that practice. Meditation, which triggers the relaxation response, was a huge boost for me.

The balance of meditation, exercise, family time, and everything else that I was previously doing, really helped. Slowly, but surely, I mostly healed from the loss I'd experienced. As anyone who has lost someone they love knows, it can take a long time to heal from these things, and even when healed, some emotions will never fade away.

Still, I was doing well enough to return to college and finished my studies with a B.S. in Physiology/Health. Due to my experience with the detrimental effects of stress and grief, I made understanding stress and how to effectively manage it a big part of my studies and academics. Stress management became such a big topic of interest for me that I even wanted it to be a part of my career. So part of my role as a Certified Health Coach has been to help people identify their top stressors and then to find relief in these areas.

In my personal life, I've also made a real commitment to living a healthy, balanced, and *truly* fulfilling life. It is my hope that you too embark on this journey in order to experience how good life can be with less stress and greater balance!

Part 1

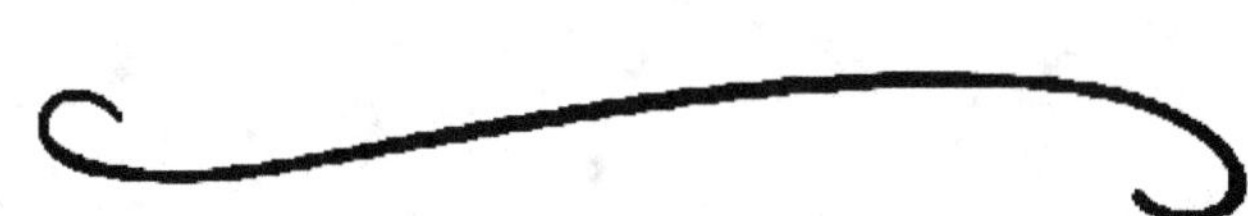

The Power of Stress

Overview

Every person wants to live a good life and to be happy. What determines whether or not a person feels happy, and what it means to live a 'good life' varies from one person to the next. Some people want to live a life that is slow and simple, with excellent health. Others want to live a fast-paced life with an abundance of money, and some people will want both good health and money together. There are many variations of what living a 'good life' looks like to people.

That being said, no matter what living the 'good life' looks like to a person, to live it, *managing stress* will be paramount. In order for each of us to survive into old age; reach our financial, relationship, career, and spiritual goals; all while having peace of mind, managing stress will be key.

So what is stress exactly? The most commonly accepted definition of stress comes from one of the grandfather's of stress research named Hans Selye. He defined stress as "the nonspecific response of the body to any demand for change." I like to simplify this definition a bit. For the sake of understanding, we will say that **stress is any action, event, or circumstance that throws the body, mind, or emotions out of a state of balance**. Usually if one of these elements goes out of balance, such as the emotions, the other two will follow.

The fascinating thing, which you will soon learn about stress, is that while it has a bad reputation, it isn't necessarily a 'bad' thing. Some forms of stress can actually be either enlivening, or strengthening, in the long run.

In terms of stress, the body basically has three modes of functioning: eustress, distress, and relaxation.

Relaxation is experienced when the body is close to a state of calm homeostasis, or balance. Relaxation is normally rejuvenating and healing, especially if a person is accustomed to being in a state of high alert. Then there is eustress. Eustress is a type of stress because it pushes the body out of balance, but it is generally enlivening and health-enhancing in the appropriate doses (more on this later). Finally, we have distress. This is what people are most often referring to when they casually use the word "stress." When distress occurs, the body usually experiences some level of wear and tear. If the distress is short-term, the body can rebuild and become stronger. This gives credence to the saying, "what doesn't kill you makes you stronger." Trees and plants will often grow stronger from enduring a thunderstorm, for example. Problems don't arise until distress becomes either long-term or chronic. This creates a situation where the health of the mind and body can become diminished.

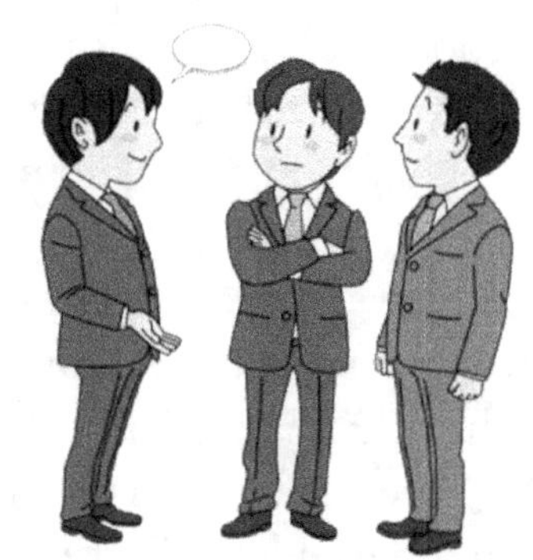

"Management is concerned, boys. One of our office plants just signed up for the stress management workshop."

Many American's have experienced the condition of chronic distress at some point in their lives. Some find themselves there currently. The good news is that there is a myriad of strategies that a person can implement to reduce their levels of distress and many of these are easy to learn, easy to practice, and don't take a lot of time.

The other good news is that our bodies are excellent at healing and repairing. The body is constantly working to heal, repair, and rebalance from the three categories of stress that affect it: physical stress, environmental stress, and mental/emotional stress.

Our **sub-conscious brain** is constantly trying to maintain a state of balance or **homeostasis** for the body. The sub-conscious brain balances our temperature, blood sugar, heart rate, breathing rate, blood pressure, etc. and generally does an excellent job of doing so. If left on their own, our bodies will generally do a fantastic job of maintaining balance. That is why animals in the wild don't get diabetes or heart disease. Their sub-conscious brains keep their bodies balanced, and when the sub-conscious brain needs help maintaining balance, the animal will feel a call to action to balance themselves. A simple example of this is a cat resting when tired. The tiredness that the cat feels is a signal to rest and restore. Bears in the wild have even been observed digging up and eating roots that they needed for medicine.

This is not to say that animals aren't under certain **stressors** and never die early. As mentioned earlier, stress is any action, event, or circumstance that throws the body or mind out of a state of balance. Animals in the wild are often subjected to the very harsh elements that they live in, and as such, can experience a great deal of **environmental stress**. Extreme cold, for example, can cause an animal to fall out of balance and possibly die.

Why is it then, that while we as humans have largely escaped the elements with our elaborate shelters and central heating, that we still so often feel out of balance? I mean, the same sub-conscious parts of the brain that keep wild animals in a state of balance, also exist in humans. Why is it then, that humans often suffer more negative health concerns and feel more uncomfortable?

This is because human beings have a **conscious/ thinking mind**. We have evolved the ability to think a much larger variety of thoughts than animals, and this *can be* an amazing gift. With our conscious minds we can dream and imagine, we can form social structures, we can remember joyful memories, and we can create. On the other hand, we can also use our conscious minds to worry, to ruminate on negative experiences, to feel regret, and to create imaginary monsters in our heads. We can also use our thinking minds to override the natural instincts that tell us to rest and restore.

Thoughts of worry, guilt, and ruminating on negative experiences all lead to a form of stress that animals really don't have (other than some living with humans) called **mental/emotional stress**. This type of stress, when strong or persistent enough, can really throw the body out of a state of balance, and even lead to illness. You may remember a time in your life where you were going through an experience that challenged you emotionally and lead to you feeling 'sick'.

Constant **mental/emotional stress** can also lead to addiction, emotional eating, verbal violence, and even more destructive behaviors. "In fact," says addiction specialist Dr. Gabor Mate, "in most cases of addiction, the addiction itself is not the problem, the addiction is an attempt to escape the problem. The real problem is often some form of physical or emotional distress or discomfort."

The reason that animals don't have mental/emotional distress in the same way that we humans do, is because they have a much narrower range of thought, and live predominantly focused on the present moment. They are neither caught up worrying about the future, nor ruminating on the past. As one wise man once told me, "For this reason, you will never find a cat with a headache!"

In today's world, headaches and chronic stress have become all too common. The world is changing fast, and at times, people feel like it's hard to adapt to this changing pace. On top of that, technology often makes it less likely for people to gather for face-to-face human interactions. These interactions always acted as an excellent buffer against stress in the past.

Another interesting thing about stress, is that when what is called the **stress response** is triggered, men and women will respond to stress slightly differently. Men will often have a tendency to either withdraw from the situation or to get aggressive. Women, on the other hand, will have a tendency to move past this 'fight or flight' response and to comfort and support the people around them. This has been coined 'tend and befriend' behavior. A man's response to stress definitely served him well in prehistoric times when there were constant threats from predators and enemies; but in today's world, the 'tend and befriend' behavior that women are more likely to demonstrate, is superior in almost every instance.

Before we discuss more on these topics and go into how a person can relieve and better manage stress levels, let's clearly define the challenges that we face in today's world regarding stress:

Challenges

1. Using the conscious/thinking mind to help us manage stress, rather than worrying, ruminating, or **'catastrophizing**.'
2. Effectively adapting to life in the rapidly changing Digital Age.
3. Using technology to our advantage rather than letting it rule our lives.

4. For men: being able to seek social support during times of distress.
5. For women: being able to find and ask for help when they have all the responsibilities of home, family, and work.

These five challenges of living in today's world are very common for people to experience. My friends, and the clients I have met with, will often bring them up. It's somewhat comforting for me to realize that while our lives are all unique, the things that we go through- our pains and pleasures, joys and fears- are quite similar.

Stress: The Good, The Bad, and The Ugly

The word 'stress' generally has a negative connotation for people. When asking a friend or loved one how they are doing, you may have heard them say, "I'm feeling stressed out from work." Or, "College can be so stressful."

You knew when you heard these statements that the person was not experiencing a positive reaction to their circumstances. This type of stress is what physiologists, who study the function of the body, call **distress**. Distress occurs when a situation is perceived to be outside of a person's ability to positively handle that situation and has negative health consequences. If a distressing situation continues, and the distress can not be overcome or better adapted to, then a condition of **chronic stress** is said to be present. Chronic stress can last anywhere from several weeks to several years.

Eustress is the term that physiologists use to describe *positive* stress. Remember when I said that situations of stress throw the body out of balance (homeostasis)? Well, imagine a time in your life where you felt really excited or challenged in a meaningful way (like performing well in a competition or planning for a big event). This situation certainly threw you out of balance, but it did so in a *positive* way.

Situations that can throw the body out of balance in a positive way vary from person to person. The same event can cause *eustress* for certain people and *distress* for others. Read this list of events that normally cause a *positive state* of stress for people and consider your own:

Positive Stress

- The excitement you felt when waiting for a band you like to step on stage.
- Dancing with friends into the late hours of the night.
- Skydiving (not my personal 'cup of tea')
- Having the person you feel attracted to give you a kiss.
- Having an uncomfortable conversation with a coworker that ends positively.
- Witnessing the birth of a baby.

All of these events can yield pleasure, enjoyment, a positive sense of self, and boost your health in the long run.

Exercise is another activity that causes stress, but can be very positive in the long run. Exercise is a repetitive movement that we engage in to improve the fitness of the body. Exercise is also done to improve the condition of the heart and lungs and can have many other physical benefits. It can even improve one's mental health. Exercise certainly places stress on the body because it raises your heart rate, breath rate, and wears on the muscles, but done correctly exercise can be a very beneficial form of eustress.

> Eustress is pronounced "You-stress." You can think of it as stress that is good for YOU.

Stress in the form of meaningful challenges that we are capable of accomplishing can even lead to a state called **flow**. Flow is a very positive, even coveted, state to be in. Going into the flow state causes performance to skyrocket. In the flow state an individual feels a warped sense of time. Time either appears to slow down or just 'fly by'. An individual in this state will also be very present and in the moment, and their sense of individual self may vanish. Athletes call this state 'being in the zone.' Jazz musicians have termed it 'being in the pocket' and say that when it occurs, good music just flows out of them spontaneously.

The types of challenges that cause an individual to enter the flow state will vary from person to person. In the U.S., **yoga** has become popular because it triggers the flow state for some individuals while they are doing the stretches. For others, more intense experiences are needed to trigger flow, such as racing automobiles. I have witnessed servers in restaurants looking very excited, and likely in the flow state, as they run around attempting to meet all of the challenges 'on their tray.' For others, this same situation will put them in a state of distress.

The bottom line is, the situations that lead to positive stress and also trigger flow, are different for each of us. We must perceive the challenge we face to be meaningful for sure, and we must also have the skills and resources to meet the challenge. If we don't enjoy the challenge, or if it is overwhelming, then distress results. If what we are doing doesn't challenge our level of skill then boredom and apathy are almost certain to ensue.

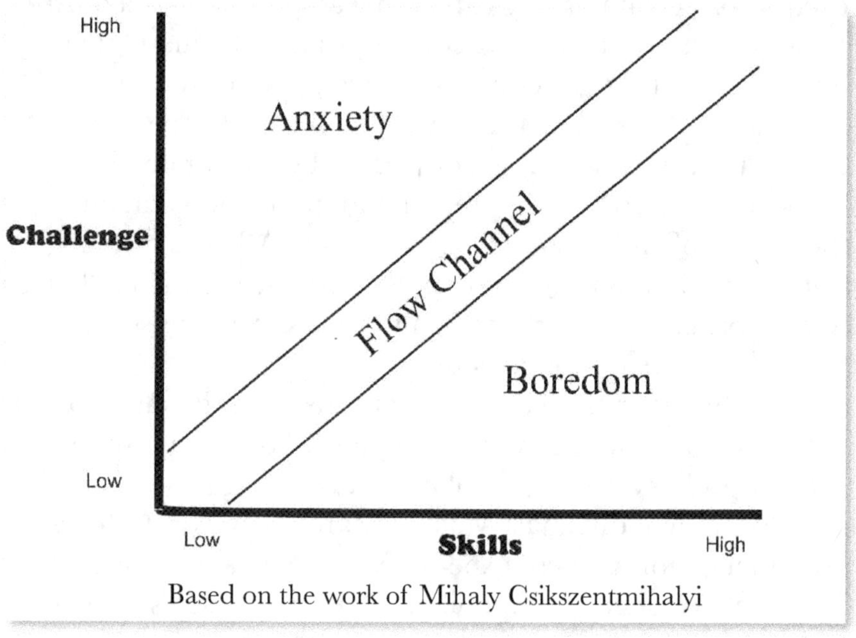

Based on the work of Mihaly Csikszentmihalyi

Top Tips for Experiencing Flow

Flow is a topic of study that one psychology researcher, **Mihaly Csikszentmihalyi** (Me-High Cheek-Sent-Me-High), has dedicated much of his adult life to studying. He has found that going into *flow* both greatly enhances one's performance and enjoyment of the present moment. He also discovered that what going into the flow-state feels like is described nearly the same by all people no matter their race, gender, age, or geographic location. If you can go into flow more often, you will likely enjoy your life more, and be able to spend less time in distress. Here are some tips based on flow research that can help you to get there:

1. Pick activities that are either pleasurable or that you really enjoy doing. This will vary from person to person.
2. Choose activities that engage you either mentally or physically with all of your attention. This is the reason

that people so often enjoy playing sports or engaging in online gaming. Gaming and sports engage one's full mental or physical capacity and have a clear goal (to either win or beat the level).

3. Have a clear goal in mind when doing activities. This can even be applied to typically 'boring' activities such as cleaning the house. Gather up your family or roommates and set a goal to clean the place as fast as possible, for example. You may find that it becomes more engaging and enjoyable.

4. Take care of your mind and body. If you are exhausted or worn out, it will likely be more difficult to experience flow.

5. Incorporate music. Even the most mundane tasks like cleaning and organizing can gain flow-potential with the right playlist of tunes.

6. Create something new. Creativity is very engaging and triggers activity in parts of the brain associated with flow states.

Three Categories of Stress

The stress that the body must deal with generally comes in three different categories. They are termed 'stress' because they throw the body out of balance in either a positive or a negative fashion.

Physical Stress

This type of stress is experienced when an activity or force acts upon the body and creates the need for repair or rebalancing. Negative forms of physical stress include things like injuries, falls, improper use of the body, and foods that cause digestive upset.

The deep-fried foods that make a big portion of the Standard American Diet are actually physically stressful, because they create inflammation in the stomach lining which takes energy to 'fix' and rebalance.

Physical stress can be positive in the form of exercise or stretching because these activities increase the tone of the body overtime. Cardiorespiratory exercise (ex: running) is a physical stress that improves the functioning of the heart and lungs. On the other hand, if exercise or movement is done improperly, it can lead to injury or physical damage (physical distress). As with all things, physical stress should be administered in healthy ways and in moderation.

Physical stress can also arise from physical trauma or an accident. Examples of this would be a baseball player getting 'beamed' by a baseball, or a person getting in a high-speed wreck. Yikes!

Environmental Stress

How healthy is your environment? Do you live in a smoky city or do you live in a fresh wilderness setting? How clean is your water? How clean is the food you eat? These are all factors that can play a <u>major</u> role in your overall stress level. Every form of environmental stress creates an imbalance in the body which the body must then use energy to correct.

Environmental stress can be accrued from the pollution of our environments which enters the body through the food, water, and air that we take in. For many people living in noisy or polluted cities, environmental stress can place major demands on the body.

An example of the ill-effects that environmental stress can cause is the fact that individuals who work with synthetic chemicals have been found to have a higher incidence of cancer. The molecules in the chemicals put stress on the body and undermine immunity.

The health of our environments is very important and taking measures like filtering water, eating organic food, and going out into natural environments to relax can all reduce your environmental stress load.

Mental/Emotional Stress

This category of stress is probably more closely associated with the word 'stress' than any other form. In casual conversations, if a friend uses the word 'stress' they are likely referring to some mental/emotional *distress* that they are experiencing.

The reason that mental and emotional stress are not two separate categories is because you can't really separate the mind from the emotions. Thoughts and perceptions are almost always the triggers for how a person feels emotionally.

All events and situations in our lives enter the mind through the senses. The mind then perceives and interprets each event as either bad, good, or neutral.

If an event is perceived as neutral, then very little change will occur in one's emotional state. If an event is perceived as *good*, then the emotional state of an individual can be enhanced and feelings of joy, happiness, or elation can occur. This is an example of eustress which is often an emotional experience.

A perception of things as *bad* can lead to emotions such as sadness, disgust, or anger. If what is being perceived is seen as both bad and threatening to either one's sense of self or one's survival, then the 'fight or flight' mode will be triggered. This will rev-up the body to act, and to deal with the threat effectively by either fighting or fleeing. If the threat is not dealt with effectively, or if a person keeps believing that they are under threat, then mental/emotional distress will begin causing serious imbalance within the body.

To have moments of mental/emotional distress is no big deal if perceived threats can be dealt with effectively, but if they are persistent, then the wear and tear on the body can lead to physical or mental illness.

The mind is a very powerful tool. Begin looking at it as such. Just like technological inventions such as computers and cell phones are tools that can be used wisely to enhance life, so can the mind.

Many sources of mental/emotional distress are virtually unavoidable. Say, for example, you see a loved one having trouble swimming and potentially drowning. You will go into the 'fight or flight' mode as a response to save them, and this mode will enhance your physical abilities of doing just that.

Mental/emotional distress can also be caused by the great transitions in life that we all go through. I had a conversation with one of my apartment neighbors in the summer of 2019, and I could see that there was sadness in her posture and on her face. I asked her how things were going for her. She informed me that she was going through a really hard time, because her husband ha suffered a heart attack one night while they were eating dinner, and he passed on. I let her know that I was really feeling for her, and I wished her well. What she told me was on my mind for many days afterward.

For a person in one of these situations such as a partner loss, divorce, job loss, or another major life change 'hard feelings' are basically inevitable. There's nothing wrong with that, and it certainly doesn't mean that there is anything wrong with that person. Hopefully, if you find yourself in one of these situations, you will look to access as many healthy resources as possible, so that you can go through the transition process with as much grace as possible. Our bodies have even adapted a mechanism for coping with the pain of loss in these situations… crying.

While there are many cases of mental/emotional distress that are virtually inevitable, there are also many-many instances of mental/emotional distress that are really up to perception.

If you go through a break-up, and you were really hoping that things would work out between you and this person, you can feel sad and distressed. On the flip side, if this person was getting 'on your nerves' and they kept you awake all night with their snoring, then the break-up may come as a relief.

Many events in life can cause one person to feel distressed and another to feel neutral. Some people are very calm in the face of challenge and others feel super anxious.

We likely all know at least one person who seems addicted to constant worry, and therefore, distress.

Just like anything, with willingness and practice we can become better at certain skills. Staying calm, relieving distress, balancing stress levels, and becoming more resilient to life's transitions are all skills that can be learned and built upon. I have seen it happen many times.

Two emotions that are commonly related to distress are anger and fear. Anger comes about when we feel like our boundaries have been crossed. This emotion can be used either constructively to give us awareness and lead us to expressing our needs productively, or can lead to destruction. Fear is triggered when either our physical survival is threatened, or when we feel a threat to our dreams, desires, and aspirations (sense of self). Both of these emotions can trigger the 'fight or flight' mode. The sooner we are able to resolve emotions of fear and anger, the sooner we will be able to move into, and enjoy, the present moment.

Our relationship with past, present, and future is also a big part of our mental/emotional stress levels. Learning how to make peace with the past, present, and future is such an important part of living life, that these concepts are a big component of many spiritual traditions.

In Christianity, for example, it is said that one must forgive the mistakes of themselves and others in order to make peace with the past. Forgiveness is a beautiful gift when one can offer it to both ourselves, and others.

In Zen Buddhism, practitioners are urged to accept the present moment and the constant change of life as a way to make peace with things as they are.

Other traditions teach that one must trust in God or the Universe so as not to feel overwhelmed or anxious about the future.

My uncle Charlie likes to live with the motto, "Learn from the past, prepare for the future, but enjoy the present." Having a positive relationship with the past, present, and future can be very rewarding, whereas a negative outlook on past, present, or future is going to be distress inducing.

If we want to make the most out of our lives, we must commit ourselves to accepting the present, forgiving the past, and trusting the future to work out for us. This is much easier said than done, but people often naturally improve in these areas with age and experience.

Pandemic Stress

As of this writing, it is October 2020 and for much of this year the world has been caught in the midst of the Covid-19 pandemic. This has created what I would say is a worldwide spike in distress levels as people are feeling more stressed from worrying about illness, feeling concerned about loved ones, and from worries about the future.

This stress is very mental/emotional in nature but can have a physical component if one does fall ill.

I would say that it's certainly good to be cautious of illness, especially as it relates to the Covid virus. I would also add, that since worry and distress can be so debilitating, it's good for a person to cope with and relieve this distress as much as possible.

If a person does realize that they are feeling a lot of pandemic stress, I would encourage them to seek out all of the healthy resources for facing fears and worries. This may include things like counseling or therapy, journaling, or talking to loved ones about concerns. It's best to talk with people who are not in a frantic state, as this may be more harmful than helpful.

Chapter 3 ~ Three Categories of Stress

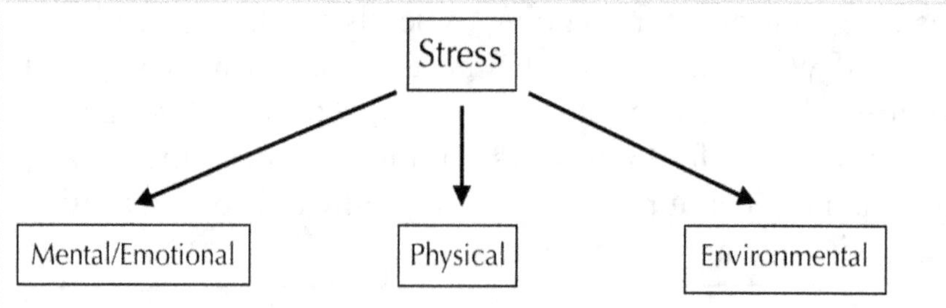

Mental/Emotional	Physical	Environmental
Distress • Failing an exam • Pulled over for speeding • Receiving bad news • Feeling insulted • Loss of friend(s) • End of a relationship • Nervous about a big event • Losing a job • Being late for work • Things not working out as desired/hoped for • Family member falls ill	**Distress** • Physical injury • Suffering a fall • Extreme heat/cold • Bad posture • Eating unhealthy, spoiled, or burnt food • Excessive alcohol consumption • Hard drug use • Whip lash • Sun burn	**Distress** • Breathing in pollutants • Cigarette smoke • Acid rain • Inhaling fumes from paint or household cleaners • Polluted drinking water • Tornadoes, hurricanes, powerful storms • Being improperly dressed while outdoors
Eustress • 'Falling in love' • Lively conversation with friends • Feeling socially supported • Overcoming a challenge • Receiving help/guidance • Accomplishing a goal • Feeling spiritually connected • Experiencing Flow **Relaxing** • Prayer/Meditation • Reading and Writing	**Eustress** • Receiving massage • Chiropractic adjustment • Welcomed sensual touch • Hugs • Proper exercise • 'Runner's high' **Relaxing** • Gentle stretching • A warm bath • Laying still	**Eustress** • Enjoying a beautiful day • Entering a fun setting **Relaxing** • Breathing in clean air • Drinking clean water • A clam, peaceful setting • The sound of waves, birds, or a soft rain

Table 1: The three categories of stress; with examples of eustress, distress, and relaxation that are associated with each category.

The Stress Response

Whenever we perceive that there is a threat in our environment- either to our physical body or to our sense of self- the **stress response** is triggered. The stress response is a mechanism that is very important to the survival of both humans and animals as a way of helping us to overcome threats. The triggering of the stress response puts us into a state nicknamed the 'fight or flight' mode.

When the 'fight or flight' mode is triggered a surge of **adrenaline** is released into the body. This causes a rise in heart and breath rate, an increase in pointed focus, a surge of sugar into the blood, and for the energy and blood of the body to go to the arm and leg muscles for action.

You know that you are in the 'fight or flight mode' when your heart rate rises and your mind begins to race. If you are really aware, you will also feel your breath getting shallow, and your muscles tighten. You are now more prepared to deal with a threat. Let's go back in time for an example:

Imagine it's the year 10,000 B.C. You're walking through a moderately dense forest with two of your tribesmen. You are either a young man or woman carrying a spear with a very sharp point. It is your job to protect the other two tribesmen, who are hunters carrying bow and arrows. The bow and arrows they are carrying are good hunting tools but are not very speedy in the instance of a predator jumping out. You know that there are rumored to be tigers and panthers in this forest.

Everyone is on high alert as you trek through the forest searching to find a deer that one of the hunters has shot with an arrow. There are blood spots on the ground; each spot being about five feet apart, and the fresh color of the blood indicates that the deer is likely not far away now. You continue to follow the trail.

As you push back some eye-level branches and walk into a clearing, you spot the deer. The clearing is small (ten feet by ten feet) and the body of the deceased animal is lying right next to some bushes. You feel excited and relieved, as this kill will be able to feed your small village for a couple of days.

But then terror strikes because a tiger jumps out from behind one of the bushes with a "Rawwr!"

Here's 400 pounds of raw fury looking you right in the face.

Immediately your heart races. Your senses heighten. You jump back a little as you lower your spear. For you, the 'fight or flight' response has been triggered. You don't have time to sit down and make a decision whether to run or stand your ground, but you do know that everyone is counting on you. You have also been taught that if you run from this, you may end up being the large cat's appetizer. So you stand your ground. You are breathing so hard that you instinctually form a circle with your mouth and breathe in and out heavily.

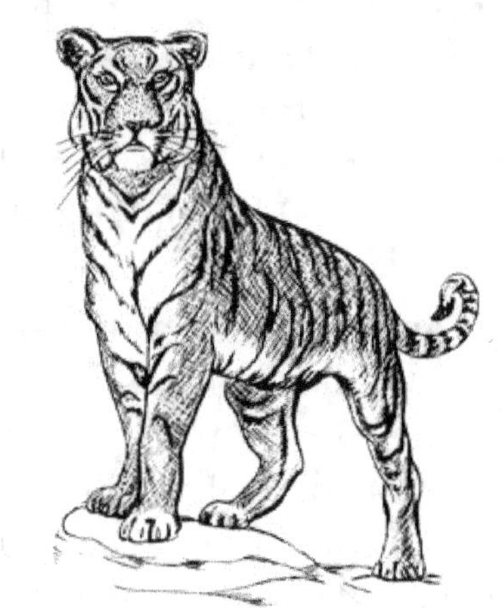

The tiger roars again, "Rawwr!" but you've already decided that you're not going anywhere, and the tiger begins to sense it. For the tiger, you see, is also in the 'fight or flight' mode.

Wild tigers are very intelligent and (s)he has an instinctual understanding of what a human being is. As part of the tiger's instincts, *(s)he knows that human beings are an apex predator and even recognizes that you are holding a weapon.*

You let out a yell, "Ahhhh!" as the tiger paces in front of the deer. Your comrades behind you draw their weapons. The tiger has sensed a serious threat and now determines that it is better to either pick another battle or to find it's own food. It knows that it can't outrun you while dragging the deer, so it retreats into the forest at a jog.

You feel some relief, but you are definitely still in the 'fight or flight' mode. Together, you and your comrades retrieve the deer and walk back to the village on high alert.

…You are now back in the village and back to safety. The walk back with the deer was tense, as you now better understand the dangers of the forest.

There is lively happiness all around you. Everyone is excited about your hunt, and the story of your bravery and courage is shared with everyone.

You get pats on the back and happy looks. The feeling of safety from being back home causes your heart and lungs to slow back down. You feel at ease. Another bodily state, which is essentially opposite to that of the stress response is being triggered: the **relaxation response**.

The above story illustrates an example of the threats our ancient ancestors faced. The tiger was an external threat that lead to the release of adrenaline and the triggering of the 'fight or flight' mode.

While many humans in developing countries must still face very real challenges to their survival, the threats that we as humans face in the 'developed world' tend to be more mental/emotional in nature. Let's look at this example:

Your name is either John or Janet, and you are driving to work. You live in a bustling city and traffic is hectic today. The hectic traffic puts you on high alert. It's a Monday, and you are hoping to get a good start to the work week. You get to work and prepare your desk. There are several other desks around yours in a large room and you have a job as a financial something or other. Your friends don't really remember what it is that you do exactly.

You look up and see your supervisor walking over. You already feel tense, remembering some of the tasks that they have assigned to you in the past. He walks up and drops a large stack of papers on your desk. He looks at you and says, "Hey, I know this looks like a lot, but we are really making a push right now as a company to get ahead, and we are giving everyone on this floor a large stack of stuff to analyze by Friday. I need you to analyze all this stuff and write a ten-page report; due to me by Friday." He then walks away.

You feel your heart immediately race. You look at a few of the pages, hoping that perhaps a bunch of them are just blank pieces of paper. Nope. It's some dense financial hoopla.

You aren't sure if you can manage to get everything done by Friday. You have your 45-hour workweek, but you also have commitments to your friends to uphold, and you don't want to work extra. You feel a bit disheartened but get to work anyway.

Your heart races and your breathing becomes shallow every time you remember the challenge of the deadline, but you continue on. This job for you doesn't stir much passion, but you feel you must do it to get by. You go home after this Monday and feel wiped out. You lay in bed with all your thoughts still stirring and wonder if you will be able to accomplish your work duties for the week.

What is happening here is that you are in the 'fight or flight' mode. You don't feel it as strongly as the villager did while defending themselves from a tiger, but it's definitely there. If you can't manage to trigger the relaxation response then you may not get to sleep anytime soon.

Unlike the villager from 10,000 B.C., you also don't have the same social support to assist you. If you stay in the stress response for too long, it may have detrimental effects on your mental and physical health and wellbeing, but you continue on doing the best you can.

This story illustrates a 21st century problem that has become all too common- too much mental/emotional distress. We as Americans are spending too much time in the stress response and not enough time in states of positive stress or relaxation. The cost this is having on our health is tremendous.

The mind and body are not separate. Every mental state that we are in (such as stress or enjoyment) triggers a cascade of hormones that affect the functioning of *every single cell* of our bodies. Due to this fact, many physical ailments are caused by too much stress, which leads the cells of the body to run in *overdrive* until they are exhausted and can't function properly. The health costs of mental/emotional distress are calculated to be in the hundreds of billions of dollars annually just in the U.S. This money accounts for the missed work time due to stress-induced illness, medical costs from illnesses caused by distress, and from costly mistakes made under distress.

Most of the stress we are now experiencing is triggered by our own minds perceiving a threat. The saddest part is, many of these threats are truly *imaginary*.

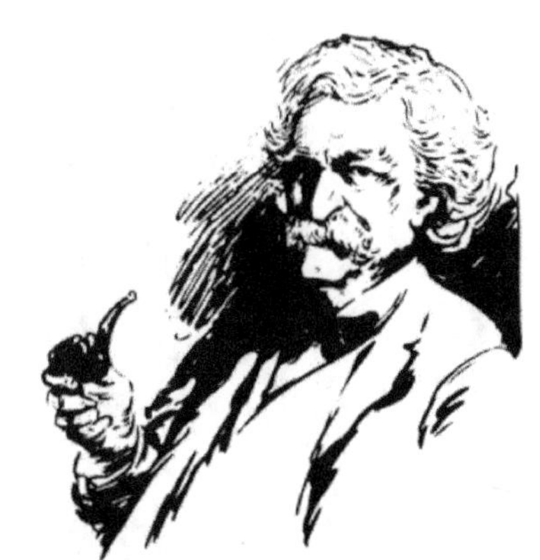

Think of a time in your life (5 to 10 years ago) when you were under a perceived threat. Maybe you were worried about running out of money and eventually being homeless. Or maybe you were stressed about a final exam. Or Maybe you had a perceived enemy to argue with.

Many times, we imagine threats outside of ourselves to be more threatening than they actually are. Many times what we fear, such as getting evicted, never actually happens. Other times, what we fear does happen, but it isn't as devastating as we had expected. This is a big reason why the older generation (65+) doesn't report experiencing higher levels of stress over the last 40 years. They have gone through enough experiences to realize that most things which people fear are just 'imaginary tigers'.

*Go to *Appendix A: The Anatomy and Physiology of Stress Management* if you would like more detail on the stress and relaxation responses. (Page 201)

The Evolution of Stressors

As previously mentioned, the forms of stress **(stressors)** that we humans face, and the stressors that animals face, can be quite different. Also, we as a human race are constantly evolving and our forms of stress (stressors) are evolving with us.

Take for example our hunter-gatherer ancestors. They experienced many of the same environmental stressors that wild animals do. They had to constantly adapt to the seasons and the changes in the weather and climate. If food was short, they would have also experienced some mental/emotional stress in the form of worry.

Hunter-gatherer life, which occurred mostly from 2 million to 8,000 years ago, no doubt had its challenges, but people living in hunter-gatherer societies also experienced many benefits from living life at a much slower pace than we do in today's world. Hunter-gatherer individuals also had a closeness within groups and tribes that could serve as a natural buffer against stress.

Then the first agricultural revolution took place. The first ag. revolution took place around 10,000 years ago (8,000 b.c.). It involved families and tribes transforming from hunter-gatherers to crop farmers. This new way of life made food acquisition much easier and cut down on hunger. This 'small farm' lifestyle was generally low on negative stress, other than during times of war or famine, and was the way of life for most people until about the 1900s.

When the 1900s rolled around, a second agricultural revolution took place (the green revolution), which marked the great movement of people from 'farm life' to towns and cities. The 1900s ag. revolution was a time marked by greatly improved agricultural production from improved farm equipment and technology. The John Deere tractor, for example, made doing fieldwork much easier and lead to more food production. The tractor also allowed an individual farmer to farm much more land.

An individual farmer now being able to farm more land, meant that fewer farmers were needed. This created a situation where some people were pushed off of their farm land and forced to adapt to town or city living. For some individuals, this was a great stressor, and for others, it was a blessing.

Around the same time that the green revolution took place, a major industrial revolution also occurred (1870 to 1920). This revolution (called the second industrial revolution) was a time when machines like the steam engine and automobile came into being. Factories began to be built, and the conveniences that people needed for daily living were pumped out en-masse. This caused many people who were working by hand such as cobblers, blacksmiths, seamstresses, and bakers to lose their jobs. A machine could now do their job much faster and cheaper than they could. Losing a job is a stressor that almost anyone would feel, and then when these same individuals were forced to work in dangerous 20th century factories, even greater stressors were experienced.

The creation of factories also brought with it new forms of air, water, and environmental pollution. Toxic chemicals were released into the air from the burning of fossil fuels. The waste products from factories were dumped into rivers and lakes. These toxic substances eventually get into the human body, even today, and cause us a modern form of environmental distress.

In the late 1900s, a new revolution began - **The Digital Revolution**. Computers, words processors, the internet, and automated services replaced many of the technologies of the industrial revolution. These new inventions also created entirely new social systems, industries, and careers. This revolution also carries with it the opportunity for each of us to make our lives easier and simpler, as long as we can learn to use technology wisely.

I remember being a young boy and going on road trips with my family to see our aunts and uncles across the state. After driving for hours, actually finding where our aunts and uncles lived in a bustling city seemed almost impossible. All we had to work with was an address and some directions scribbled on a spare piece of paper. One adult would be holding a map and yelling at the driver to turn either to the left or to the right. Us kids would become anxious from all the uncertainty and start to complain and yell. It was chaos.

Nowadays, when my family and friends go on trips, we have Google maps to guide us. We can just type our destination into an application and be directed there seamlessly. We don't have to worry about getting lost anymore. Just like this example illustrates, we can all use technology to help us find our way through life. On the other hand, if we are not conscious about how we are using technology, it can also create more stress in our lives and take us prisoner.

One of the things that the digital revolution often does, is force people apart. It makes it so that we can do so many things 'on-line'- such as work, play, shop, and communicate- that we often don't go out to see people as often for face-to-face interactions. The face-to-face human interactions and social gatherings that have always been apart of human history gave each person an opportunity to share in their joys, struggles, stresses, and strains; and come together to support one another.

The **blue zones** are areas of the world where people routinely live to be the age of 100 more than anywhere else. A commonality of many of these 'blue zones' is that the people living in these areas are constantly surrounded by a circle of close friends and family. Having a strong social support network, no doubt, helps a person to better manage stress and to live a longer and happier life.

Another challenge of our digital age is the pace at which life is constantly changing. This, for some, can trigger stress and anxiety. It can be hard to keep up with the constant changes in the economy, new products, and constantly evolving careers.

In our digital age, we must all face the challenge of using technology as a tool to make us healthier, rather than sicker. If we can each dedicate ourselves to finding new ways to use technology positively and to help us gather, then we can effectively adapt to the challenges that the Digital Revolution presents.

Short-Term vs. Long-Term Stress

As stated previously, whenever we experience a perceived threat to either our physical survival or to our sense of self, the stress response is triggered. When the stress response is triggered, adrenaline is released into the bloodstream in less than a second. Adrenaline wakes us up and causes us to feel more alert. We are immediately more focused and our heart rate can either increase or sky-rocket, depending on how serious we perceive the threat to be.

Adrenaline 'fires us up' and gets us ready to either 'fight or flee'. The release of adrenaline doesn't tend to last for very long, though. After that, if we can find a way to handle our stressor, then adrenaline will subside and we can return to a more balanced physiological state. An example:

You are sitting in English class. You've gone through almost the entire class period without your teacher realizing that you didn't read the assigned material for last night, nor did you do a summary of the reading. There are only five minutes left of class. You are feeling good. You are gonna make it unnoticed.

All of a sudden, the teacher mentions the reading from last night. She says she'd like to hear some student feedback on the plot of the story.

You feel yourself go from calm to tense. Your hands get clammy. The teacher looks at you and it's almost as though she can see right into your guilty soul.

She calls on you to stand and give your honest feedback on the reading. Oh snap! Busted. You feel the adrenaline coursing through your veins now. Your heartbeat is so loud that it can almost be heard by the student sitting next to you. In this scenario, you have an especially strong fear of public speaking and you don't want to be embarrassed. You perceive a threat to your 'sense of self' taking place, because you don't want people to perceive you as either lazy or dumb for not doing your assignment. You feel your face get hot and your hands tremble.

You stand up anyway, and say, looking down, "I didn't think that the reading last night was any good, because I didn't read it."

Everyone laughs. Your teacher, turning a bit red, but deciding to show you mercy, says that she'd like you to catch up on all of the reading tonight. You nod in agreement to her request and sit.

You feel a bit ashamed, but immediately after class a friend approaches you and cheers you up. They let you know that they thought the whole event was hilarious, and that they liked your honesty. You feel much better now, and decide to settle down.

This story illustrates an example of how adrenaline fires us up when we perceive a threat. Athletes taking the field for a championship game will feel it; auto racers on the first lap experience it; and you will feel it if a loved one is perceived to be in danger and you want to help them. The stress response, and the release of adrenaline, can be very advantageous in these ways because it focuses us in and it gears us up for action.

After the big game is over or the perceived threat we are faced with has subsided, adrenaline release slows back down and gives us time to rest and repair.

If the threat that we are facing doesn't subside, or if we continue to imagine facing imminent threats to our well-being, then we will go into a state known as **chronic stress**. Many people in this day-and-age live in a state of chronic stress as they incessantly worry about threats to their livelihood, family, or sense of self. Chronic stress can also come about from having chronic unresolved emotions like anger or guilt.

Cortisol

When the 'fight or flight' response is triggered, another hormone that plays a key role in the stress response will flood the body in larger-than-normal quantities. This hormone is called **cortisol.**

Cortisol is released by the adrenal glands that sit on top of the kidneys. Cortisol is a very profound hormone within the human body. It is in charge of feelings of wakefulness, energy metabolism, insulin release, relieving inflammation, and even plays a big role in immunity. If you imagine the food that you eat as providing your body with energy like gasoline does for a car, then you can think of cortisol as being responsible for how that gasoline is released and when it is used (sort of like a gas pedal).

We all experience a rise in cortisol levels in the morning. This rise wakes us up and gets us ready for the day. After this initial rise, which lasts from around 6:00 to 9:30 am, cortisol levels will slowly go back down until around 3 pm. Then cortisol takes a dip in it's release. You may have felt this 'afternoon dip' before. Cortisol release will also taper off in the evening
which makes this a good time to relax and prepare for sleep.

Whenever cortisol release is heightened, due to either its daily cycle or from the 'fight or flight' response being triggered, a greater amount of energy is available for usage. This is because cortisol triggers greater amounts of sugar (glucose) to enter the bloodstream. Cortisol also causes more insulin to be released into the blood, so that the sugar can be brought into the cells for energy usage. This provides us with the energy we will need to accomplish our daily tasks. When cortisol levels are 'jacked-up' during the stress response, we will also have more sugar and insulin in the bloodstream to energize us for dealing with perceived threats.

Under non-threatening circumstances here is a healthy cortisol curve:

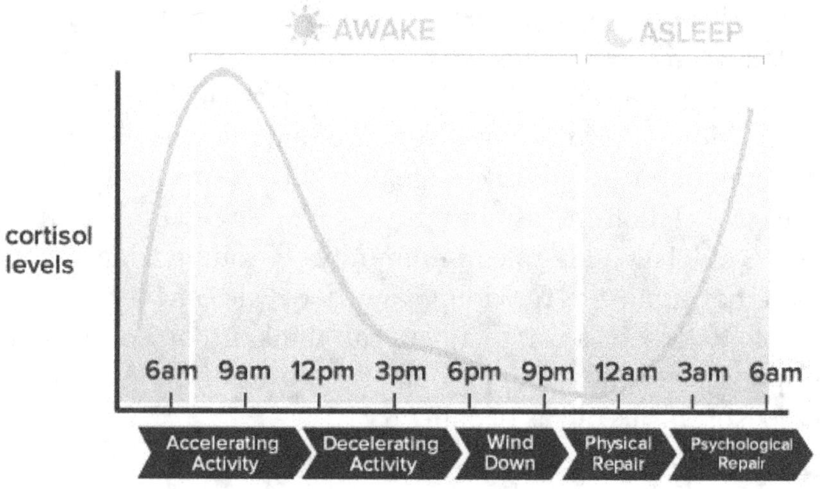

Under good to ideal conditions, cortisol will follow this natural daily cycle. This natural cycle of cortisol release is what our hunter-gatherer ancestors would have experienced on most days. They would have felt sleepy at night due to an increase in **melatonin** and a decrease in cortisol. After a good night of sleep, where there were no artificial lights, this individual would have then naturally woken between 5:30 am to 7:30 am as the sun rose and their cortisol spiked. At 3:00 pm, they would have likely rested, before returning to their daily tasks.

This is how life would have been for most people living in hunter-gatherer societies where there were not as many stressors and no technological distractions. These people's life expectancy was certainly shorter, but it was often healthier due to the balanced state of their hormones.

What is happening in today's day and age; with more artificial lighting, technological advances, and chronic stress, is that people's cortisol release has been thrown off. Under conditions of chronic stress, the body and mind are running at high speed, because the gas pedal (cortisol) is being pressed down more frequently and causing a greater release of fuel (glucose).

After a certain length of time, which varies from individual to individual, the body and mind will eventually become exhausted from running at high speed and will then 'cry out' for rest. Unfortunately, the individual who is in this state will likely reach for a quick pick-me-up in the from of sugary foods or caffeine, instead of giving their vehicle (the body) the rest that it seriously needs. The pick-me-up will last for a short time, but will perpetuate problems in the long run.

The heightened release of cortisol can eventually lead to a condition known as **adrenal fatigue**. This condition has been written about thoroughly in Dr. James Wilson's book *Adrenal Fatigue: The 21st Century Stress Syndrome*. Adrenal fatigue occurs when the adrenal glands release so much cortisol over a long period of time that they can't keep up with the demands any longer. The cortisol release then drops, because the body has essentially run low on this vital hormone.

The cortisol will then be produced and released at just a trickle compared to that of a healthy adult. This will leave an individual feeling very tired, because cortisol is too low for a healthy release of sugar and insulin into the bloodstream.

Under these conditions, it's also likely that the individual will have difficulties with chronic inflammation because cortisol is also used as an anti-inflammatory in the body. As I said, it's a profound hormone. It also has many duties.

Here is a story of adrenal fatigue (called non-Addison's hypo-adrenia in medicine):

Dr. T.W. is a professor working at a small college in Colorado. He is a black man who teaches African Studies and African-American

Justice to his students. Knowing the challenges and the difficulties that African-descended people face in the United States, he is happy to teach the subject. He can see that his students really catch on to the issues that Black people face in the United States, and often become passionate about changing things for the better. He is really liked by the students and faculty.

T.W.'s problem is that he has now said 'yes' to too many commitments in his work life, and this is having negative consequences on his overall health and personal life. He has a family with a wife and two kids with who he loves to spend time, but on top of that, he is also teaching and grading for four classes, advising, working as a political activist, and sometimes writing articles. He often spends 70-80 hours a week on work duties.

His passion for his work, which has turned into an imbalance, has now caused him to feel burnt out, and he finds himself feeling tired constantly. Every morning and afternoon he pulls into his favorite coffee place for a needed pick-me-up. What used to be one small coffee drink has now become two larges.

T.W. has many deadlines in his work life that he must meet and without realizing it, he is constantly in 'fight or flight' mode due to his fear of not keeping up with his commitments. Eventually, T.W. feels like he is just dragging himself around. He doesn't know exactly why his once abundant energy is now faltering. To add to that, his family doctor has diagnosed him with high blood pressure, and T.W. has gained 10 more pounds around his mid-section. T.W. just continues on, not realizing that the stress he is under is causing him to feel tired, and is having other negative consequences on his health.

Dr. T.W. is in a state of chronic stress leading him to feel burnt out. He first used up his adrenaline resources to get himself 'fired up' for the day of lecturing. After the adrenaline was depleted, his body began using larger amounts of cortisol to keep him energized and in the 'fight-or-flight' mode. This seemed to work well for a while, but eventually, the cortisol became depleted, just like the adrenaline before it. When the cortisol then became depleted, Dr. T.W. felt a drop in his energy, because cortisol is needed for energy release and usage.

Operating in a condition of chronic stress can eventually lead to a state of either burn-out or adrenal fatigue. It's estimated that at least 30 million people living in the United States are suffering from this condition (hypoadrenia).

<u>Hyper- Vs Hypo-Adrenia</u>

<u>Hyper-Adrenia</u> occurs when our bodies produce higher than ideal amounts of the adrenal hormones, including cortisol. These elevated levels can be triggered from being in the stress response. When cortisol is at higher levels, a person will feel energized, but a bit frantic. If these levels do not recede, then the individual will eventually feel fatigued due to the body running on overdrive. This may also cause a person to have difficulty sleeping, leading to a "tired but wired" condition.

<u>Hypo-Adrenia</u> is a condition where the body is producing lower than ideal amounts of the adrenal hormones, such as cortisol. It can happen for a variety of reasons; including chronic stress. In the field of medicine, severe hypo-Adrenia is referred to as Addison's disease and must be treated with synthetic hormones.

12 Symptoms of Chronic Stress

Chronic stress can cause a whole cadre of mental and emotional discomforts. Here I will explain twelve of the major ones, chosen mainly because of their frequency.

In truth, there are dozens of ill-effects that chronic stress can have on the body/mind of an individual. If you have a discomfort that you think may be associated with distress, do your own research on whether or not stress is linked to your dis-ease. You can pay attention to what is going on in your life when you have a physical or mental discomfort, to see if distress is linked.

Brain Fog: The stress response causes the blood in the brain to be directed to the brain's more primitive areas for quick decisions and survival. Parts of the brain needed for clarity and higher reasoning will essentially be turned off, which can eventually lead to feelings of 'haziness' or 'brain fog.'

Chronic Pain: Being in the 'fight-or-flight' mode causes the muscles of the body to tense up in preparation for a serious physical effort. This tension occurs even if the stress is mental/emotional. If this tension lasts for a prolonged period, then the muscles of the lower back, arms, and legs can feel sore. This painful situation can also extend to the joints and worsen arthritis.

Digestive Issues: During the stress response, blood and energy is diverted away from the digestive system and into the muscles and joints. Without this blood and energy, it will be more difficult to digest and assimilate food that is consumed. It also makes it more difficult to maintain the digestive tract lining. Even the best food will not benefit the body as much during times of chronic stress, because the nutrients that are in the food will not be digested and assimilated as well.

Fatigue: During the initial stages of distress, a cascade of hormones including adrenaline and cortisol is released to energize the body for action. Staying in this state for too long eventually causes the cells of the body, which have been working in overdrive, to feel exhausted. Remaining in this state can also lead to low cortisol levels, which is needed for proper energy release and usage.

Headaches: It's well documented that stressful situations can contribute to migraines headaches. Since migraine headaches are difficult to treat with medication, it's crucial for migraine sufferers to reduce or eliminate stressors. Another class of headaches- tension headaches- can also be worsened by stress, especially the stress caused by loss and grieving.

Hypertension: Chronic stress raises blood pressure and can lead to an increased risk of hypertension (chronic high blood pressure). Stress can also be a leading cause of more serious heart conditions.

Inflammation: Inflammation is created in the body when the immune system is trying to heal the body from some type of damage. You may notice when you have a cut that the area around the cut becomes red and puffy. This puffiness is inflammation. Inflammation will also occur in areas where the body is attempting to remove invaders.

When people have seasonal allergies, the nose and eyes often become inflamed as the body is attempting to remove invaders (allergens) that it believes to be threatening. Cortisol, which has the job of energy distribution, is also used to counteract inflammation in the body. A synthetic form of cortisol, called *hydrocortisone,* is often used in allergy medicine. Under the conditions of burn-out, a person's cortisol reserves will be lower. This means that when people are burnt-out, there is less cortisol available to counteract inflammation. This can exacerbate the symptoms of allergies and/or lead to chronic inflammation.

Insomnia: It's impossible to turn a car off when it's still in gear, unless the engine faces adversity and dies. So too, it's very difficult to fall asleep if your mind and body are 'still in gear.' The stress response revs-up your body and mind for action (puts them in gear). Getting out of the 'fight or flight' mode must be achieved for optimal sleep or possibly to sleep at all.

Lowered Immunity: During the 'fight or flight' response, the energy and blood of the body is diverted to the muscles and joints for immediate action. This causes energy and blood to be diverted away from areas of the body in charge of immunity such as the liver, kidneys, and bone marrow. As such, chronic stress can lead to repeated colds and sinus infections.

Moodiness: Chronic stress can lower levels of the 'happy hormone' **serotonin**. This in turn leads to a feeling of agitation, anger, and a negative outlook.

Reproductive Issues: Being in distress lowers a person's chances of becoming aroused, and lowers sperm count in men if the distress is long-term. Think about it, if your body gears you up to fight for your life in the 'fight or flight' mode, what are the chances of you wanting to 'make love.' A period of mental/emotional distress can also worsen symptoms of a woman's menstruation.

Weight Gain: Chronic stress can lead to weight gain in two ways. Firstly, when individuals are under distress, they have a tendency to reach for sugary foods as a way to keep the body running at a high level of activity. During times of high stress, you can expect the lines at coffee houses to be long, as people reach for these sugary and caffeine-laden drinks to keep themselves going.

The second way that chronic stress causes weight gain is through the release of insulin. Insulin is released in higher proportions during times of chronic stress which causes extra fat to be stored in the belly region. If an individual has extra belly fat compared to the rest of their body, then chronic stress could be a contributor.

Distress Load

What is your level of physical distress? Feel free to pull out a piece of paper and a pen and give your physical distress level a ranking from 1 to 10. Then rank your mental/emotional distress from 1 to 10, followed by your environmental distress. Add the three numbers together and this could give you a good idea of your overall distress level from 0 to 30.

Distress is additive and cumulative, which means that all the stressors in our lives come together to form our overall stress level. Every form of stress we experience creates a demand that our systems must deal with.

Stress levels tend to be different from person to person and fluctuate with the changes in our lives.

From my research, I feel strongly that physical, environmental, and mental/emotional stressors are major contributors to most illnesses and diseases. Mental/emotional stressors can be major contributors to mental illness, such as anxiety and depression. Overall chronic stress can lead to physical ailments. In regards to illness, diet, exercise, mental outlook, social health, age, genetics, and stress levels will all be leading factors.

As you learn to better manage the stress in your life, you will find that your body and mind can both heal quicker, and feel like they are functioning more efficiently. This is because the causes of physical and mental discomforts are almost always linked to some category of distress.

<u>Distress Load</u> =
Physical Distress (Stress on The Body)
+ Environmental Distress (Pollution, Noise, Extreme Climate, etc.)
+ Mental/Emotional Distress (Negativity Around Past, Present, Future)

If you notice that you are taking on a lot of physical distress from either over- or improper-use of your body, now could be a good time to consider what you may do differently. If you commonly breathe-in either environmental chemicals or pollutants, you may be able to get a mouth and nose covering to protect yourself from these airborne irritants.

Unless you are either working with hazardous chemicals or are a professional football player undergoing the physical strain of an intense contact sport, mental/emotional distress is probably a bigger factor in your life. Mental/emotional distress, without a doubt, constitutes most of what we experience as *distress* and discomfort. In parts 2, 3, and 4 of this book, we will cover how to better manage this type of stress in deep depth.

Individual Differences

How each person reacts to an external event can vary greatly from one individual to the next. In terms of stress, some people are capable of remaining relaxed throughout the ups and downs of daily living, whereas others become distressed by the slightest inconvenience. The same exact event can cause one person to feel elated and happy, whereas another person feels nervous and distressed.

If your favorite sports team scores a goal or a point, you may jump up and down and feel elated. The fans of the opposing team, in contrast, may grumble and get 'cranky.' It's the same event, but people reacted very differently based on their hopes and expectations.

While riding with different drivers in dense city traffic, I've noticed that some people stay calm and relaxed, while others get tense and 'on-edge.'

I've also noticed in my academic life that an upcoming college exam will create very different stress levels in students. Some students are well prepared and not worried about the exam at all. Others are well prepared but they have a personality that tends toward worry. Some people aren't prepared at all, but they don't seem phased. And some students will show up for the exam frightened half to death and forget everything that they studied because they are in the 'fight or flight' mode- not the thinking and remembering mode. There is a lot of individual variation in response to external events.

The way that distress affects each person's mind and body, when it does occur, can also vary considerably. Two people can have the same exact chronic stressor and the same level of stress, but the effects it has on their mind and body can be very different. For one person, chronic stress may lead to them having an upset stomach with peptic ulcers and blood in the stool. Another person may have breakouts of acne on their skin and face. For another person, chronic stress may lead to *invisible* symptoms, because their distress leads to mental/emotional illness.

In our culture, the people who feel physical symptoms of stress, as opposed to mental ones, are almost lucky because they have a way to visually prove the discomfort that they are going through. This can lead to people feeling more sympathy and concern for them.

On the flip side, if chronic stress causes mental/emotional discomforts, it would seem that people are not as likely to understand or sympathize. It is easier to take 'sick days' at work for colds and flus than it is to take them for 'feeling down.' We are just beginning in our culture to take mental health concerns seriously.

So as you see, people react to stressors differently, and people's bodies and minds respond to stress differently.

There is also individual variation in how much stress a person can handle. The same amount of stress can cause two people to collapse at different rates. One person may collapse from the same stress in two years, the other in 40.

Most people would think that a person who can go longer before collapsing under the weight of chronic stress is either lucky or more fortunate. I would disagree. I actually think that it's better for your body to give you the message that you are under too much stress sooner, so that you can then have the motivation to change your circumstances. You can use this motivation to adopt new habits that lead to greater health and happiness.

Stress and Mental Illness

Undergoing chronic stress can exacerbate, or lead to, a greater occurrence of mental illness in individuals who already have a tendency to suffer these conditions. Cortisol is released in greater quantities during stressful experiences, and scientists have found that people with depression tend to have higher than average cortisol levels.

Also, if you consider the symptoms of burn-out (fatigue, listlessness, trouble focusing, lower sex drive, less enjoyment), it would stand to reason that being chronically stressed, to the point of exhaustion, can lead to an episode of **depression**, because the symptoms of the two are very similar. Feeling distressed can first cause an individual to feel slightly depressed, as the depression in this case, is a sign that the body wants to rest. If not dealt with, the stressor can cause a more serious episode of depression from a person being more out of balance.

Mental/emotional distress can also be a trigger for **anxiety,** and chronic stress can exacerbate chronic anxiety. In fact, anxiety and the stress response can feel very similar.

The stress response is triggered by a real or perceived threat in the environment of an individual. It can make one's thoughts race and cause a host of physical discomforts. An anxiety episode is similar to the stress response in feeling.

The difference between anxiety and mental/emotional distress, is that anxiety can turn on at any moment, even if there is no known threat in the environment.

Distress can trigger anxiety in some individuals (but not all), but anxiety can also feel like it comes out of nowhere.

Stress and Trauma

Traumatic experiences are events that are so stressful that they leave a lasting impression in the mind of a person. The traumatic memory can be 'triggered' by some outer stimuli, which causes an individual to go into a strong 'fight or flight' response. The stress response from **trauma recall** can even be so strong that it causes a third reaction which is to 'freeze,' as in becoming almost immobile. When trauma is triggered, it also causes a strong experience of negative emotions associated with the trauma. An individual who has witnessed a friend die in combat, for example, may feel intense fright and sadness when even the smallest 'trigger' causes them to remember the incident.

Mental/emotional distress and trauma triggers can both put an individual in the 'fight or flight' mode. The main difference between emotional distress and trauma, is that trauma recall tends to be more powerful and uncomfortable.

In a state of trauma recall, there tends to be more emotions, and trauma triggers are often very harmless to outside observers. An individual who has been physically abused as a child may get very frightened when they hear a door slam; their brains recalling this sound occurring before their abuser attacked them. If there are six other people in the room with this individual, the other people may not feel any reaction from the slamming of the door, whatsoever.

In the scientific community, we are just beginning to realize that there are a vast amount of people walking around with unhealed and unresolved trauma. People often think of the most serious incidences of PTSD, caused by war, being what constitutes trauma, but in fact, it encompasses much more than that. Individuals are experiencing trauma from all kinds of physical, sexual, and emotional abuse. Even a small amount of abuse early on in life can cause unresolved trauma, because children and infants are at a very delicate stage of development.

Trauma can be caused by intense physical, mental, or emotional distress. The triggering of trauma throws the body into a strong 'fight or flight' response.

Identifying Your Stressors Activity

What things in your life are causing *you* distress? These are your stressors. If you would like to start lessening a stressor, there are generally three ways of doing so:

1. Better adapt to it.

2. Relieve the symptoms of the stressor outside of it. (Relaxation or Coping)

3. Eliminate the stressor.

Those are the only ways to get out of distress- you can adapt to your stressors more effectively, practice stress-relieving techniques outside of them, or remove them from your life completely.

You can work on this on your own. Pull out a piece of paper and a pen and at the top write 'Biggest Stressors.' You may find that when you reflect on it, it is easy for you to label all of the things currently causing you distress. Write them down. After identifying all of your stressors, rate their severity on a scale of 1 to 10. This will help you to realize the severity of your stressors, and if you commit yourself to reducing them, you can also look back and realize your progress.

Now that you have made your list, look at your top stressor and consider what you could do to reduce, eliminate, or better adapt to that source of stress.

Examples:

- *Mark realizes that the paint fumes he is inhaling at work are causing his lungs physical distress. He commits himself to buying and wearing a ventilator over his nose and mouth to filter the air that he is breathing.*
- *Josie is constantly annoyed with her supervisor who causes her distress by making rude comments. She decides to have a talk with him about her feelings and warns that she will get human resources involved if he does not change his behavior.*
- *Francisco has noticed himself being consistently worried about his finances. He decides to rent a cheaper apartment and downscale some of his other expenses, which he hopes will relieve some of his money concerns.*

The Power of Stress

Stress can lead to exhilaration and be a powerful force for getting us out of bed in the morning. It can fire us up for a big event and cause us to hone in.

Or stress can be debilitating. It can mobilize so many resources in the body that it eventually leads to exhaustion.

It can enhance or diminish.

The stress response is a very powerful force, and if you've read this far, I hope you can see why.

It has been my intention thus far to educate and inform you on the power of stress in a simple and understandable way. If you are one of the millions of individuals feeling chronically stressed or burnt-out, I hope you have found this information insightful. I also hope that you decide to make a commitment to living life more in balance.

The information in the rest of this book can help you to find more balance, lead you to less stress, and give you peace of mind.

I try to incorporate stress management into my daily routine as much as possible. I encourage you to do the same. The joys of living life in a state of balance, far out-weigh anything we feel that chronic stress can give us.

We must, as individuals and as a collective, commit ourselves to more effectively managing stress. This will allow us to create lives more enjoyable for ourselves and for everyone living on this planet.

Part 2

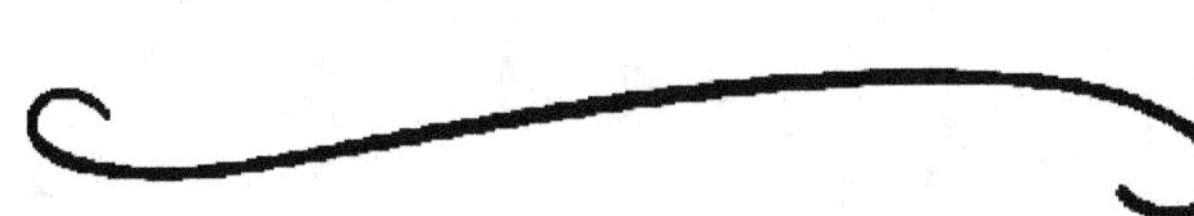

On Balance

Balance

"Like with anything in life, find the balance between too
much work and being too lazy."
-Christian Olsen

If a person wants to live a life that is full of health,
happiness, and harmony, learning how to balance opposites
will be key. To be at our best at work, for example, we will
likely need to take some time outside of work to do things that
we enjoy doing just for fun. To really show up and be at our
best in our relationships, we will have to spend some time
alone to reflect and get to
know ourselves, and to feel
healthy and vibrant, we will
have to balance the doing of
things with simply resting,
relaxing, and rejuvenating.

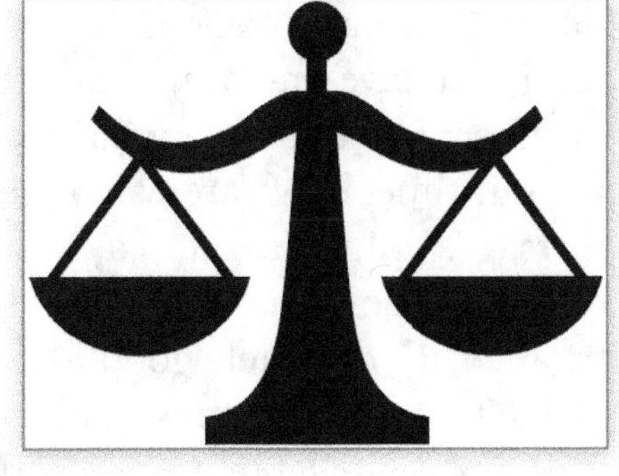

When I was younger,
I didn't understand the
concept of balance. I had
heard about its' importance,
but I didn't *get it*. I just assumed that if something was good
for you, or that if you felt good doing it, then that must mean

that the more time you spent doing that thing, the better you would feel. As such, I spent too much time in my early college days hanging out with friends, partying, 'working out,' and getting obsessed with school activities.

I had to learn the hard way that *more* isn't always *better*. I kept doing more and more of the things that I thought would bring me fulfillment, until there was a huge imbalance in my life, and I was exhausted. I didn't understand that I also needed time for things like reflection and relaxation.

Fortunately for my health and sanity, I eventually figured out how to live more in balance.

The Balance Scale

So what is balance exactly? We've all heard the term *balance* and likely we've been reminded of its importance, but what is it and how do we achieve it?

One online dictionary says that *balance is an even distribution of weight enabling someone or something to remain upright and steady*. If we apply this definition to human life, it would imply that if we wish to remain upright and steady, then we must learn to evenly distribute the "weight" of our opposing demands and needs.

In our lives, our bodies will act as the scale telling us when our time usage is out of balance. If we spend too much time in the stress response, for example, then the body will feel tired and have one or more of the symptoms of ongoing distress. The body is a great messenger for telling us how to use our time, if, we are willing to listen. It will give us messages to move, rest, play, sleep, and eat, for instance.

I believe that to fully understand the concept of balance, it's definitely good to consider the opposing aspects of life for which we must find a balance between. This table is not exhaustive but does include many of the big ones:

Sleeping vs.	Being Awake
Rest vs.	Activity
Body Relaxing vs.	Body Moving
Alone Time vs.	Time Spent With Others
Going Out vs.	Staying In
Time in Stress Response vs.	Time in Relaxation Response
Time Working vs.	Leisure Time
Time in Eustress vs.	Deeper Relaxation
Time Eating Food vs.	Time Digesting Food

It's not always easy to find a balance between our demands. If you are a parent to a large family, for example, you may find it hard to grab some needed 'alone time.'

If you have a business with several employees, then everyone may be constantly counting on you to be at work. There are many pressures that we all face, from the outside, to have our time spent in certain ways. I feel like the key to balancing our time is to make sure we are balancing time spent on our responsibilities with activities that help us to get to where we truly desire to be in life.

For example, if you are young, and one of your biggest goals is to have a loving family one day, then a big part of your time will be spent creating a strong bond with the person you want to start that family with. If you haven't met that person yet, then alternatively, you may be spending more time out-and-about meeting people.

If you look at the balance table, you may notice one or two areas of your life where you are definitely out of balance. Some people spend too much time "resting" compared to "moving" and this leads to them feeling lethargic. Music artists, who tour often, are known for spending too much time "out" and "awake" and not enough time "sleeping" and "staying in." This, unfortunately, can lead to them having shorter life spans.

If you observe the balance table above, you may also consider where we are at as a nation (the United States) in terms of balance. Its been found, in multiple studies, that many people in this country are not getting enough sleep, spend too much time sitting, and are feeling too distressed (for optimal health).

If we can learn to live more balanced lives, then our health will be greatly improved, and annual healthcare expenses will drop dramatically.

Learning how to balance the opposing aspects of life creates a situation where a person will feel healthier and more *at-ease*. Many chronic diseases that people experience develop as a result of having one or more of the elements in their lives out of balance.

For some people, it may feel as though *imbalance* is almost inevitable. Many people who have several demands pertaining to the survival of themselves and their families feel this way. Hopefully, this individual can find a way to ask for help and to outsource some of their responsibilities, in order to make time for their needs.

I have known other people who are constantly under stress in an attempt to accomplish some impressive feats, because they wanted to gain the admiration of others. I have also seen people who stress themselves out trying to uphold a near-perfect image. For these two individuals, approval-seeking has got them out of balance. These people will do well to find what truly makes them happy, because that it isn't something that comes from the approval of others.

Stress vs. Relaxation

In this book, the biggest area of balance that we are concerned with is the balance between eustress, distress, and relaxation. Both eustress and distress end in the word -stress, and they must be balanced with relaxation for optimal health and well-being.

Obviously, these two stresses are not created equal. Eustress more often occurs as a response to either fun or engagement, and distress is more closely related with fear, anger, and worry.

The thing is, no matter what state of stress a person often finds themselves in, relaxation will be needed for balanced living. It will also be needed for physical and mental healing and repair, as well as to get a good night's sleep.

Another key point here, is that while we typically think of relaxation as something done outside of work and activity, a person can actually train themselves to feel relaxed at any time. In the beginning, it will be good to have time to one's self for intentional relaxing, but with practice, relaxation can be achieved almost anywhere. I have come to notice that many of the best quarterbacks in the NFL stay relaxed when the big game is on the line, and as such, are very efficient.

13

The Relaxation Response

As you know, the body has a stress response that is triggered whenever a real or imaginary threat is perceived. In this case, the blood pressure will rise, sugar (glucose) gets released into the blood, and the energy of the body goes to the arm and leg muscles for exertion.

In human beings, the nervous system, which is basically 'the wiring' of the body, is also capable of triggering something called the relaxation response. This is very fortunate because just as chronic stress can lead to damage, the relaxation response leads to healing and repair.

For some people, watching a romantic movie triggers relaxation. For others, playing golf does the trick. Some people like to go to either a church or a temple and connect with a Higher Power to relax their minds and find a sense of peace. Whatever your choice of relaxation may be, know that relaxation is a very real state of physiological functioning that is very healing and restorative. In fact, the long-term effects that the **relaxation response** has on the body and mind are almost opposite to that of chronic stress.

Triggering the relaxation response requires feelings of safety and well-being, as opposed to perceptions of threat. Once the relaxation response is triggered, our heart rate will slow down, breathing will slow (and the breath will go into deeper areas of the lungs), a person's mood will lift, and the blood and energy of the body will go from the arms and legs to the internal organs. It's a great state to be in.

While the stress response is nicknamed the 'fight or flight' mode, the relaxation response also has a nickname- the 'rest and digest' mode. Being in this mode of functioning at night will make it much easier to fall asleep. Triggering relaxation during the day makes digestion and assimilation of food and nutrients much more efficient.

Knowing how to trigger the relaxation response causes physical healing to take place at a much faster rate, because in the 'rest and digest' mode the immune system is enhanced.

Within our DNA we have perfect instructions for how to heal and purify our unique bodies. Triggering the relaxation response allows those instructions to be activated.

Being in the 'rest and digest' mode is amazing, and it's something that, with practice, we can learn how to master as we go about our days.

18 Symptoms of The Relaxation Response

Triggering relaxation is accompanied by a release of hormones that get sent to, and positively influence, every single organ of the body. As such, triggering relaxation has a powerful effect on the body, mind, and emotions of an individual.

Staying in the relaxation response can have cumulative benefits over longer periods. Just as prolonged stress can add up and take its' toll on the body, so too, a relaxed individual will experience compounding benefits over years of practiced relaxation.

Learning to relax is an art... one that we will discuss more soon. Just know that while our culture doesn't often promote relaxation, as it does stress, triggering relaxation can be profoundly healing and truly restorative. Learning to trigger relaxation in chunks, over years, can have a lot of positive effects on a person's health, relationships, and even finances. Here are some of the short and long-term benefits of triggering relaxation:

Clearer Thinking: When the brain is under constant stress, the higher reasoning centers of the brain virtually shut down, creating a feeling of fogginess. Triggering relaxation will help the brain to turn on the higher reasoning centers (such as the prefrontal cortex directly behind your forehead) and to clear away the fog. Improved clarity of thought can also help an individual to make better choices and to know what it is that they want from life.

Feeling More Energized: Under chronic stress, the body will eventually cry out for rest and recovery, leading a person to feeling exhausted. A person who has low stress, on the other hand, will likely have more energy. The body will rebuild and repair during relaxation and the individual will eventually feel inspired to move and act.

Balanced Blood Sugar: Under relaxed conditions, blood sugar levels will return to normal as long as a non-diabetic person avoids the over-consumption of sugar and simple carbohydrates,.

Improved Quality/Quantity of Sleep: Sleep is great. Everyone who doesn't get enough good quality sleep is especially aware of that. Triggering relaxation will improve one's ability to both fall and stay asleep. Relaxation balances melatonin production, which is the main hormone in charge of feeling sleepy and falling asleep. A person living in balance will likely feel tired and want to sleep around 930 pm due to the natural daily cycles of cortisol and melatonin.

Improved Digestive Functioning: When the body and mind of an individual are relaxed, a lot of blood and energy goes to the digestive organs for proper digestion/assimilation of food and nutrients.

Greater Libido: The adrenal glands, where adrenaline and cortisol are produced, also produce many of the sex hormones. Having a balance of positive stress, a little distress, and some relaxation will leave the adrenal glands healthy and well. Healthy adrenals will produce a good amount of sex hormones and leave an individual with an enhanced sex drive (libido). If you practice relaxation, you've been warned.

Enhanced Fertility: Under times of distress, a human's interest in reproduction and ability to reproduce will go down. Think about it, if you live in a tribe of people who are under distress due to food shortage, why would you want to add another mouth to feed? Learn to relax, and your chances to create a healthy and happy baby will multiply.

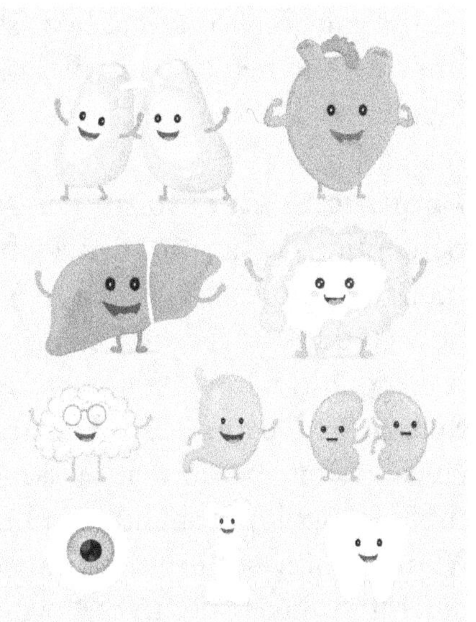

Enhanced Heart Health: Triggering relaxation lowers blood pressure and heart rate. This means that there will be less 'wear and tear' on the heart and blood vessels.

Improved Immunity: There is no single organ or location in the body where the immune system is located. There are actually many areas of the body that contribute to healthy immunity, such as healthy bone marrow, digestive organs, kidneys, and the liver. When the body relaxes from the 'fight or flight' mode, all of the immune organs will be enhanced. This makes a person better at fighting off infectious disease, bacteria, and viruses.

Faster Healing: Once the immune system is running well, a person's cuts, scrapes, and diseases will all heal faster.

Improved Performance: A person with a calm mind and relaxed demeanor will perform better under stressful circumstances and make fewer mistakes.

Elevated Mood: Triggering the relaxation response has actually been proven to increase the levels of feel-good hormones like serotonin. People who know how to stay relaxed and calm will positively influence others with their good moods.

Healthier Gut: Being in a relaxed state, either while going about your day or after the tasks of the day are over, will improve the health of your stomach and intestines. The incidence of ulcers and digestive discomfort goes down with relaxation.

Looking Sexier: In studying men's and women's perceptions of attractiveness, it has been documented in multiple studies, that both men and women are more attracted to the faces of people who look more calm and relaxed and who have lower levels of cortisol.

Stronger Bones and Teeth: Higher distress levels will cause faster breakdown of bones and teeth, and also make it more difficult for calcium to be assimilated into the bones. Many people suffering from osteoporosis have increased their calcium intake only to discover that calcium has a difficult time being deposited into bones unless stress is properly managed. Triggering the relaxation response makes it easier for calcium to be assimilated from the digestive system and eventually into the bones.

More Enjoyment of Life: Not surprisingly, if your mood is elevated and your mind is clear, you will enjoy your life more fully. Having a more relaxed state of functioning can also enhance your senses, and cause you to enjoy the 'little things' in life.

Positive Influence: As you live life with more mental clarity and calmness, the people around you will feel encouraged to do so as well. We all know what it's like to be around a person who is stressed, irritable, and tense. If this person is a manager, head coach, or a team leader, their irritability will be apparent and likely cause others to feel the same. A person who is relaxed and at-ease can have the same affect on a team but in the opposite fashion. People around this individual will feel more relaxed and calmly focused due to this person's influence.

Broadened Awareness: Being in the stress response causes our awareness to really narrow down so that we can focus on a single threat in our environment.

Triggering the relaxation response will have the opposite effect. When we feel relaxed and at-ease, our awareness can broaden and take in more of the sights around us. Picture a person sitting on a bench and enjoying a sunset, for example. This person's awareness will be simultaneously taking in many sights and sounds. Really mastering relaxation can even have somewhat of a spiritual component, as it's been theorized that a person's awareness can feel so broad that they may feel more expansive and connected to something larger than themselves. Triggering relaxation with the tool of meditation has been said to trigger states of *bliss* and unity within one's environment.

Optimal Balance

So which is better to experience- the stress response or the relaxation response? Okay, it seems kind of obvious at this point.

But before we go on condemning the stress response, remember that it functions for our survival. Not only that, but a little bit of stress is actually a good thing. A small amount of wear-and-tear can lead to a stronger self in the long run.

So far, we have discussed the stress response and how it is triggered, the relaxation response and how it is triggered (with more to come), and we have also learned about eustress.

So how much distress (negative stress) is good for us?… This will differ from individual to individual.

How much eustress (positive stress) is good for us?… We are capable of enjoying quite a bit.

How much time in the relaxation response is good for us?… A sense of relaxation will hopefully be included in as much of the day as possible. Deeper states of relaxation, which we can experience in many ways, can also be beneficial for the mind and body.

Recipe for Optimal Stress

	Distress (Fight or Flight)	Eustress (Positive Stress)	Deep Relaxation
Examples	Running Late, Being Angry, Feeling Rushed, Getting 'Triggered' or Significant Losses	Enjoying Friendship, Moderate Exercise, Sexuality, Watching a Good Movie, Planning a Fun Event	Calm Breathing, Sitting Outside in Peace, Listening to Calm Music, Reading
Ideal Percentage of Your Week	1% to 10%	20% to 80%	10% to 50%

The above table is an estimate of the percentage of time one should spend in each mode of functioning during the week for optimal balance. There will be a lot of individual variation in this matter. The bottom line is, most Americans spend far too much time in the distress mode and not nearly enough time in the other modes of functioning.

Contemplate how much time you spend in each mode of functioning. Then consider ways that you could bring more of an optimal balance to your life. Are there fun and engaging activities you could take part in, so that you can enhance your time spent in eustress? Are there activities you already know of that can help you to trigger deeper experiences of relaxation?

Resilience

Resilience, simply put, is an individual's ability to handle, cope with, and bounce back from the difficult experiences in life. According to the APA, "Psychologists define resilience as the process of adapting well in the face of adversity, tragedy, threat, or significant sources of stress."

Any improvement you make in your ability to manage or relieve stress will boost your resilience.

Some people seem to be born with a more resilient personality than others. Other people develop resilience through repeated setbacks or significant loss. Either way, resilience is certainly a personality trait that can be learned and developed.

The 6 pillars of this book are essentially methods a person can use to develop their resilience. Resilience often takes a bit of creativity, acceptance of one's circumstances, self-care, and is assisted with a *light-hearted* attitude.

When life gets very challenging, it can take a lot of courage to keep going on, and to overcome the challenge. When a person does overcome a daunting challenge, they will develop resilience, and be more prepared for subsequent challenges.

There are several amazing instances of resilience in the face of stress and challenge that have occurred within the human race. One notable resilient hero is author Viktor Frankl. Mr. Frankl was a prisoner in Nazi concentration camps for over three years during WWII and experienced almost unspeakable hardships and losses. Still, Mr. Frankl managed to both survive and hold onto hope until the concentration camps were finally liberated.

He was even able to find some meaning and purpose to his life, while in the concentration camps, where he often did his best to give hope to other prisoners. He also held on to the belief that he would one day be liberated and write about his experiences. No doubt, holding onto hope and finding meaning in the midst of his immense stress and suffering, is what kept Viktor Frankl alive. He later wrote about his experiences in his book *Man's Search for Meaning*, which became an international bestseller.

Even though we may not go through the same level of distress that someone goes through in a Nazi concentration camp, it's worth respecting that day to day stressors, or the difficult distress that loss brings, can leave us feeling like we are prisoners in our own lives.

Stories of great resilience like Mr. Frankl's (you may know some of your own) can help us to realize the strength of the human spirit and to know that we too will make it through our struggles. Resilience is a trait that can be learned with hope, willingness, and an ability to find meaning in our lives- even from our suffering. With time, you too will grow in resilience and be able to find meaning in the difficult events of your life.

Balance and Goal Attainment

For a person to even want to live life with more balance and less distress, there has to first be a desire to do so. This desire is often born from some level of discomfort or suffering. A person then decides that a change has to be made. A cry goes out within the depths of their mind and soul to feel better and to return to health and well-being. Since you have gotten this far in the book, it's likely that you either wanted to master the concept of stress management, or are one of these people who are under chronic distress and wants to return to balance.

Recovering from burn-out is something that anyone is capable of. It's also possible to live a fulfilling life that includes work, friendship, and financial prosperity; all while feeling healthy.

The Connection Between Stress & Goals

The stress response can be triggered when our survival is threatened, but it can also be triggered when we perceive a threat to our **sense of self**. That is why people are often so afraid of public embarrassment and public speaking. There is a fear here that they may be so humiliated that they will never be *seen* the same.

When a person's **goals** are under threat, especially if that goal is very meaningful for an individual, intense frustration can be experienced. In this case, it is likely that the stress response will be triggered to a lesser or greater degree. This is because a person feels a threat to who they are, or should be.

Having our goals challenged from the outside, and experiencing setbacks, is a pretty natural part of life. The path between where we are now and where we would like to be is never without some obstacles. Troubling experiences can happen in our personal lives that make goal attainment challenging, things can change, or the world around us can even transform all together. This is part of human life.

The people who experience setbacks, and then re-think a way to achieve their goals, are the ones who we most often admire. You may know somebody who, no matter what life throws at them, is able to bounce back, and even make something positive out of almost any experience. Having this kind of mentality leads to qualities of *perseverance* and *adaptability*.

At other times, when we experience setbacks, it may cause us to rethink our goals in a way that either gives meaning to the setback or is more in alignment with our true heart's desire. Some individuals who are raised in a challenging and poverty-stricken environment, for example, eventually make it their mission to help others growing up in those same neighborhoods.

Having our goals derailed or hampered can cause us stress. The reverse is also true. When we are under a lot of stress, it can cause us to have a difficult time moving toward our goals. Those are the two reasons that the concept of desires and goals are included in a book like this. There is a close connection between stress and goal-attainment.

If you are going through a time of upheaval in life, for example, it can be a source of great mental/emotional distress and lead to nagging health concerns. These nagging discomforts then make it more difficult to focus upon, and move towards a goal.

Sometimes in life, the best measure for us to take when we are overwhelmed with stress and we feel stuck, is to just slow down and take care of ourselves. Maybe for you, that means more rest, more time spent with loved ones, or slower eating habits. Experiment with the best **self-care** practices for your unique self, and don't be afraid to ask for help when you need it. Your goals will still be awaiting you when you return to better health. In many cases, self-care can also be the best measure an individual can take for moving towards their life's vision.

Being in a good state of health will often be a big part of an individual's true desires, and therefore, should be included within your vision for your life. Sometimes, people have goals that they feel are so important, they end up sacrificing almost everything, including their health, to get there. What they will likely discover, is that almost no goal is worth sacrificing their health and well-being for. In fact, the reason we feel **heartfelt desires** and set goals in the first place is usually to feel better being alive.

Desires: The Big 5

While we all have unique desires, there are generally 5 areas that almost every person's desires fall under. It's one of the things that makes us all human and all very equal. After all of our basic needs are met- for water, food, physical touch (with self or other), shelter, and comfort- we will all receive urges to follow more expansive desires. Here are the 5 categories our heartfelt desires will fall under:

Work ~ This involves finding a purposeful way to spend our time or a way to fit into our communities. It is also associated with the next desire.

Finances and 'Stuff' ~ We seek financial prosperity for many reasons. Some of the popular ones are: safety, freedom, fun opportunities, and to have nice stuff.

Health & Appearance ~ We almost all have certain health goals that involve looking and feeling better. Sometimes illness and discomfort is what it takes to awaken us to the importance of health and wellbeing. As the adage goes, "health is wealth."

If we have pain or discomfort, we would prefer it to go away. If we feel sad, we will likely want to be happier. If we feel like the condition of our body is unattractive, we may desire to make it more attractive. (Hopefully, this last one doesn't become an unhealthy obsession).

Relationships ~ Every person wants to have a good amount of trustworthy friends. It's also true, that at some point, almost everyone seeks companionship with a romantic partner.

Connection With a Higher Power ~ The reason there are so many temples and churches in the world is that most people want to connect with something greater than themselves. For spiritual aspirants, this can become their top desire.

Your Unique Vision

All people desire to experience certain things in life. Some of these desires are very momentary or seem to derive from a sense of what other people tell us that we *should* want. Desires like these tend to fade away with time.

Other desires seem to come from a place deep inside of us and end up only growing with strength over time. I like to call these *heartfelt* desires. I use the word 'heartfelt' here, because anyone who is well connected with their 'inner world' will understand that the heart basically has an intelligence all its own. There is even a lot of scientific evidence of this, as it's been discovered that within the heart there is an elaborate network of neurons (brain cells).

A healthy adult will take the heartfelt desires they feel, and create *goals* to help themselves pursue, and hopefully experience, these desires. These are what I call the *ultimate goals,* and they come together to help create a unique vision for how a person wants their life to be, or to turn out.

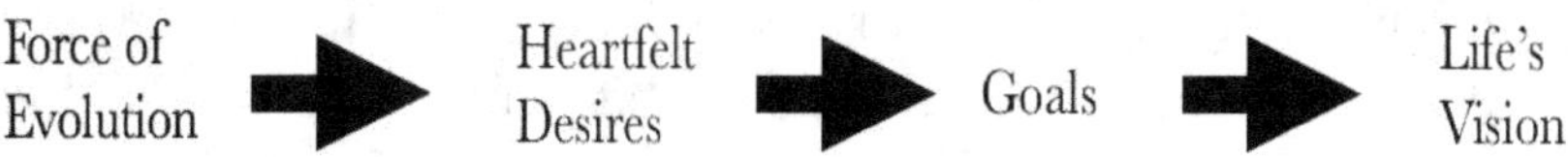

Everyone will have a slightly (or very) unique vision for how they want their lives to turn out based on their ultimate goals. And that's okay. No person's vision is right or wrong- as long as it is something true for them.

We all have a force inside of us that is pushing us to evolve, to expand, and to seek greater levels of harmony. We see this force acting everywhere in nature- in species, in communities, and in individuals. I believe that this force is what causes us to birth our true, heartfelt desires. These desires arise from the force that is pushing us to evolve and expand.

When we follow the urgings of this force, our desires will lead us to greater happiness, health, and fulfillment- all things which improve our likeliness to survive, prosper, and create greater order within our environments.

At times in life, we may have to choose to follow our own heartfelt desires, even though other people want to influence our choices. I truly believe, that if we are true to ourselves and follow our heartfelt desires, we will also be doing what is best for everyone around us. This is because we will be healthier, happier, and more evolved in the long run.

We also have a force within us that causes us to choose actions based on fear alone. This force pushes us to simply survive for the sake of surviving and can keep us in the *stress response*. We must learn to acknowledge whether or not we are choosing actions based solely on the need to survive, or if we are following the desires that push us towards greater harmony and happiness.

There is nothing wrong with working and acting for survival, but if our life becomes totally consumed with these activities, we should stop and consider how we would like our lives to *ideally* turn out.

True heartfelt desires support greater happiness, health, and harmony, and are good for all the living beings around us. They give us a sense of purpose and lead us to having a better chance to survive as a species.

Honor your heartfelt desires, and create your goals based on these yearnings. Here are a couple of examples to consider:

Margaret is a business executive who has been called into a meeting at work. She walks into the room where the meeting is being held, and finds that there are already twenty other people gathered in the meeting room waiting for an announcement. The company president stands up and announces that there are going to be some promotions.

One of the bigger promotions ends up going to Margaret. People clap and applaud while looking at her. This is a great honor, but inside Margaret feels uneasy. She knows that her true desire is to hopefully get married to her fiancee, Jim, within the next year and to then start a family.

The promotion she received will make it more difficult for her to take time off of work to be pregnant and raise her beloved children.

Johan is a chemistry major at a state university. He hails from Central America and it has been his dream to get a degree in a U.S. college since the age of 15. He is so close now...

He is working on his final paper for his senior project and then "OH NO!" His computer dies and stops working. The paper he had written is lost forever. It's a devastating blow, but he decides to hop on another computer and start again. He is not going to let anything stand in the way of his academic goals.

Tenzin and Jampa are Tibetan twins that grew up in China. They have now reached the age of 19 and are leaving the family home to seek their own path in the world. Tenzin is a more introverted individual who enjoys traditional Buddhist meditation practices and chooses to join an order of monks. He tells his brother that long days of meditating cause him to feel a great sense of peace, and that he can use his peaceful presence to influence the world positively. Tenzin wants his brother Jampa to join him.

With some hesitation, Jampa joins Tenzin for a week of meditation and service to others. The long hours spent sitting in meditation lead to Jampa feeling utterly bored. He can't understand how Tenzin can handle this drudgery. Jampa doesn't realize it yet, but life is calling him to evolve in a more worldly fashion.

In the case of the twin brothers, you can see how two individuals who have so much in common- like twins- can have very different desires. Neither of their desires (or goals) are bad. Tenzin is attempting to bring more peace to the world, and Jampa will explore what his path of evolution is, out in the world.

Goals & Balance

No matter what your goals are, it's unwise to pursue them so fervently that you forget about balance. In one of the examples above, the devout-Buddhist monk named Tenzin was spending long hours in meditation. It will be important for this individual to remember both the importance and the value of connecting with others, not just his 'inner self.' When I was in college, I had to learn the importance of balancing activity with much-needed rest.

The balance of how much time we spend doing certain activities will be influenced majorly by what our goals are. We all have the same amount of hours in a week (168) to spend.

Margaret, in the example above, was not as thrilled over her promotion as some of her coworkers would have been, because she wanted to shift the balance of her life towards more family time.

No matter what your heartfelt desires and goals are, it's good to realize that if these two things do not match, it is hard to feel your most satisfied and inspired. For example, if deep down you desire to dance and paint more in your life, but all your goals pertain to owning a nice house and working a lot, with no consideration of dancing or painting, then you will feel some uneasiness.

It is also true that we are all slightly (or very) unique in our desires. A good friend is one who will respect your true heartfelt desires, and be able to tell you when they notice what most excites you and makes you come alive. That is one way to tell when you've found a true heartfelt desire- to see what excites you and makes you come alive!

Stress and Personality

    How we approach the accomplishing of our goals and the pursuit of our desires has considerable individual difference. Some folks will push ahead no matter what is in their way, and they will do so in an effort to accomplish their goals as quickly as possible. I like to call these people **strivers**. They are constantly *striving* to better their lives and are very driven. Sometimes, these people cause themselves a great deal of distress in the pursuit of their dreams and goals.

    Other people have more of a relaxed and easy-going approach to life. They see life as more of an adventure, an experiment, or a ride. They live more with a present-moment focus and enjoy the sights and sounds that surround them. For this reason, I would call these people **present-moment-enjoyers**. Present-moment-enjoyers are more likely to enjoy their lives *now*, rather than later. They are more likely to work as artists, actors, or talk therapists, whereas the strivers are more likely to get into business, sales, or management.

    Understanding our **personality** can be very helpful for understanding who we are, what we like and dislike, and whether or not we tend toward being either stressed or relaxed.

While it's true that each of us has a unique personality, there are certain personality types that we all fall into, which we can learn more about in order to gain insight into our tendencies.

In the field of Psychology, they have identified four personality groupings that every individual falls into based on their attitudes, behaviors, expressions, and moods. These personality types are labeled Type A, Type B, Type C, and Type D for easy reference. Each one of us will tend to express different elements of the different personality types at different times in our lives. That being said, there will likely be just one (possibly two) personality types that we most identify with. This personality type (or two) will influence our predominant mode of expression for the rest of our lives and also influence how we approach the pursuit of our goals.

Each personality type has certain strengths and weaknesses and tendencies towards either balance or imbalance. That being said, a person can achieve balance and peace no matter what personality they have. Learning what your personality tendencies are through self-awareness can help you to take advantage of your strengths and better adapt to your weaknesses.

Read through the personality types and see which one(s) you connect with.

Personality Types

Type A

The Type A personality is the striver that I mentioned above. Type As like to be in control of themselves and their environment. They like to delegate to others at work and can be very passionate about what they do. They are the personality most likely to be described as perfectionists. **Perfectionism** is a quality that is occasionally admired in the world of work but can also have negative consequences. The perfectionistic quality is likely to lead to Type As putting too much pressure on themselves and others, for example.

The identifying of Type A people has become so popular that calling people 'Type A' has even made it into popular culture.

This group is the one most likely to burn themselves out with distress. This can happen when they *strive* for success so hard, whether it be in relationships, finances, or at work, that they wear themselves thin. Some scientific research has even found Type As to be the ones most likely to suffer from heart disease.

On the positive side, it's also been found that there are many successful people with a Type A personality that aren't burnt-out. Type As, in fact, can be quite good under pressure.

Any person can learn to accomplish their goals without burn-out, IF they can manage stress effectively. If you are a Type A individual, the advice in part 3 of this book will hopefully help you to effectively manage your stress levels.

Type A (Striver) Weaknesses	Type A (Striver) Strengths
• Overly-Competitive	•Takes Charge
• Easily Angered	•Passionate
• Abrupt	•Ambitious
• Impatience	•Can Be Good Speakers
	•Self-Motivated

Type B

People with a Type B personality are the least likely to stress themselves out in the pursuit of their goals. This group is most likely to get their sense of fulfillment from what is happening around them *now*, rather than waiting for fulfillment in the future. This is the group that I referred to as the present-moment-enjoyers above.

Type B individuals usually have a relaxed and easy-going type of functioning. They are usually very social, and people often love the way that they approach life. While they are relaxed and like to enjoy the present, they can also get excited and energized if they are with a group of people they enjoy.

Where the Type A personality will often pursue very worldly and practical ventures, Type Bs are more likely to record songs, get involved with planning events, and making art.

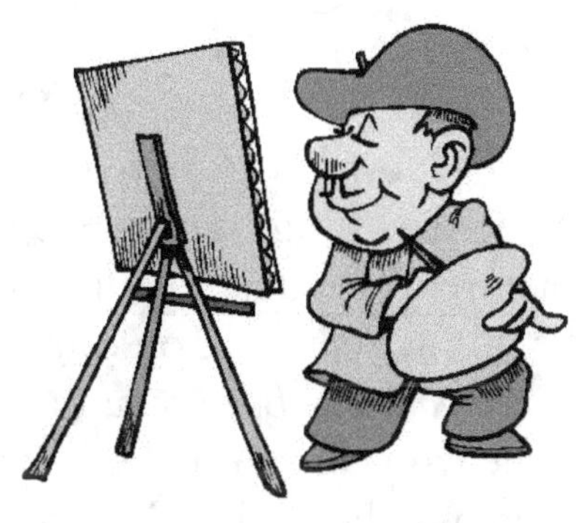

People with a Type B personality are the least likely to be over-ambitious in the pursuit of their goals and the most likely to be patient. That being said, no one is immune to stress, and anyone can experience the troubling effects that living in the fast-paced United States can have. Type Bs are simply the least likely to get swept away by it. If you have a close friend who you feel has a Type B personality, my suggestion to you would be to spend time around them in the evenings and on the weekends so that they can help you to relax and unwind.

Type Bs biggest weakness (and possibly their biggest stress) is that they can be **people pleasers**. People pleasers will often go to great lengths to make others like them, even when it has negative consequences. If the people in their lives take advantage of this fact, then the Type Bs may experience stress from people placing a lot of expectations on them.

<u>Type B (Present-Enjoyer)</u> <u>Strengths</u>	<u>Type B (Present-Enjoyer)</u> <u>Weaknesses</u>
• Good With People	•Poor Time-Management
• Enthusiastic	•Can Get Distracted
• Creative	•Attached to Being Liked
• Light-Hearted	•Can Take on Too-Many
• Relaxed	Things (Due to Enthusiasm)

Type C

Now to the Type C personality. Psychologists recognize this group of people as ones who tend to be 'big picture' thinkers and enjoy time spent alone solving problems or simply reflecting on events. If you have seen the movie *Beauty and The Beast*, you may remember the main character Belle who constantly had her "nose stuck in a book." Then there was her father, Maurice, who was constantly inventing things. These are two good examples of Type C characters.

We can nick-name this group 'thought lovers.' Thought lovers often enjoy very practical matters like the Type As, but they also enjoy thinking outside of the box and considering all possibilities. Unlike Type B individuals, they like to spend time alone and are more introverted.

Examples of professions that Type C individuals are drawn to include: engineering, computer software design, and physics. They love theories and seeking solutions through careful thought. In decision-making roles, they will look at all sides of an issue before coming to a conclusion. They will also have the facts to back up their conclusion, once it is reached.

The Type C personality will approach stress management with an open mind and look to solve their problems either on their own or with self-help resources. They can be good at coming to solutions to almost any problem and following through.

The Type Cs biggest issue with managing stress is not knowing when to ask for help and being too withdrawn. Not knowing when to ask for help can force an individual to take on too much on their own. Being withdrawn can leave a person without enough social support.

Still, if we can learn to understand ourselves and our traits, we can find ways to adapt to, and overcome, any of our weaknesses.. For Type C personality individuals this will look like getting out of their comfort zones to seek good people for help and support.

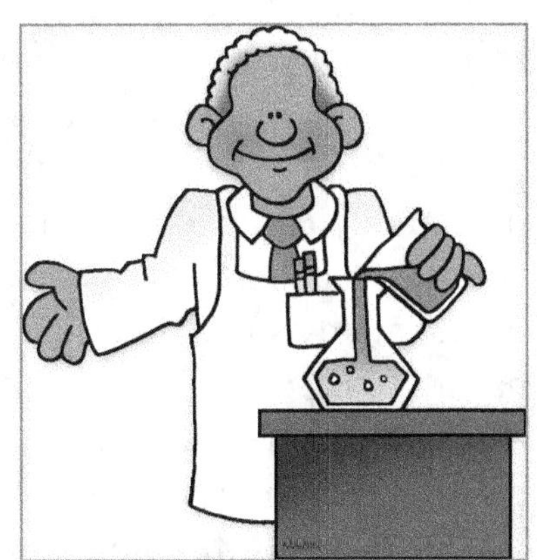

Type C (Thought Lover) Strengths	Type C (Thought Lover) Weaknesses
• Accuracy	• Withdrawn
• Imagination	• Critical
• Detail-Oriented	• Avoidant of Relations
• Intelligent	
• Curious	

Type D

The last personality grouping that Psychology has identified in regards to stress is the Type D. We will call these individuals the 'stable' group. This is because they are often slow-moving, slow to change, and very routine. It's common for people with this personality type to also carry a little extra weight on their physical bodies, due to their slow-moving and stable nature.

The 'stable' personality type is often a very caring group (that can make good caregivers). They enjoy making peace with those around them and being gentle with others. They are often calm and grounded.

People with the Type D personality can become good social workers, teachers, counselors, and financial advisors. Their caring nature makes them comfortable to be around. They are often trustworthy and reliable.

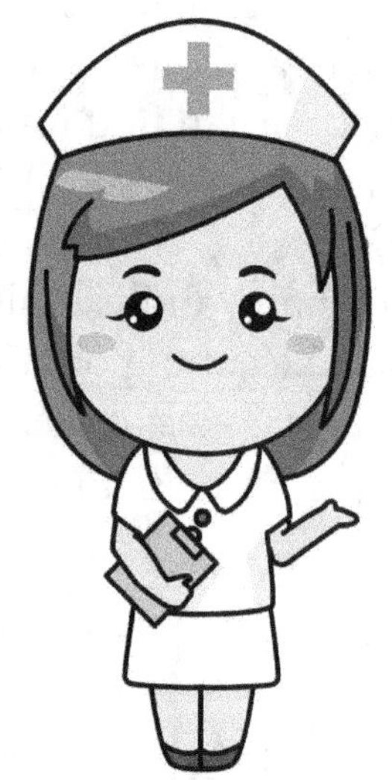

Type Ds main personality weakness is that they can get 'stuck in a rut.' That means that when they get into a routine, it is often very difficult for them to change that routine, even it is not serving their desires or goals.

Type Ds are also the personality type most likely to feel helpless or hopeless if they don't know how to make their desires come into their lives. At times, Type Ds can feel depressed if they can not experience what they really want. They often don't have the same drive and 'fire' as a Type A individual.

Type As can get burnt-out with too much fire, and Type Ds can become stagnant with too little.

Still, Type Ds are very good people to have on a team and often bring a very calming presence. They don't mind repetition, and for this reason, they can master tasks.

A good health strategy for Type D individuals is to exercise often so that they can enliven their steady-moving nature.

Type D (Stable) Strengths
- Caring
- Calm
- Trustworthy
- Consistent
- Even-Keel

Type D (Stable) Weaknesses
- Resists Change
- Slower Moving
- Holding Things In

Self-Awareness

Understanding who we are as individuals- with all of our unique strengths, weaknesses, attitudes, and tendencies- can help us get the most out of life. In life, self-awareness is key. As the sign above the oracle at Delphi says, "Know Thyself."

We all have strengths that we can draw from. We also have weaknesses, which, if we can become aware of, can actually be used to our advantage. The Type A individual, for example, may choose to make several Type B friends, so that they can have people in their lives that help them to enjoy the present. They may already be drawn to that type of person without even realizing it. A Type D individual may seek out a Type A individual to have on their team, so that they can feed off of that person's fire and determination.

We all have personality tendencies that we receive from our environments and our genetics. I believe that each of us also has innate personality tendencies, which will naturally reveal themselves if we allow ourselves freedom of expression. This means, that deep down, we all have ways of thinking, being, and acting that are unique and true for us. Eminent Psychologist, Dr. Carl Rogers, coined a term for a person who has their thoughts, beliefs, words, and actions all in alignment. He called this person a **congruent** individual.

When we stay true to who we are as people and express ourselves congruently, we have a greater chance of being happy and healthy. This is because what we *feel* we want, what we *say* we want, and how we *act* are all in alignment. If we try to force ourselves to be a certain way to fit into a situation, then we will likely feel some discomfort and unease.

If we express ourselves authentically, then we can begin to see how we tick, and how we can best respond to stressful situations.

Enjoying What Is

Do any of the four personality types seem relatable to who you are as a person? I personally recognize myself as mostly a Type A individual, and have struggled with the annoying consequences of perfectionism in my life. One of the reasons I've found myself so personally interested in stress management is because I feel like it's easy for a Type A person, like myself, to want to achieve all of their goals quickly and to stress themselves out in the process.

Through self-awareness and a lot of reflection, I've come to realize that while attaining goals is great, it's not what makes life deeply fulfilling.

The 'high' that someone experiences from attaining a meaningful goal tends to be very short-lived. I now believe that our greatest opportunity for happiness in life is by learning to enjoy the present moment *just as it is*.

Moving in the direction of attaining one's goals, then, is best when it's done with the intention to enhance one's enjoyment of the present. Moving towards a meaningful goal can be a great way for us as people to feel excited, creative, and optimistic about what's to come. It can also boost our confidence and skill.

I believe that a great recipe for acting and living is this: **We enjoy life as it is, while also moving towards more fulfillment.**

A lot of people who seek the accomplishment of their goals through intense striving and struggle, actually delay their joy until they acquire what they desire. This leaves them putting a lot of stress and pressure on themselves as they pursue their desire fervently. The problem with this attitude is that even if this person does attain their goal, they will normally not enjoy it for long. This individual has made a habit of struggling to accomplish something at the expense of the present and will likely just create a new goal to struggle for.

Being truly happy and enjoying the present are skills that take practice. They don't come from the outside world.

If you have heartfelt desires that you want to experience for yourself, then move towards them, and do so with commitment. But while you are on the way to getting what it is that you feel you want, don't forget to enjoy life, just as it is. Perhaps along with financial, relationship, and status goals; also set happiness goals. This will help you to open up to the things that help you to be happy *now*.

Maybe there are people you love being around whom you could spend more time with. Or maybe you want to explore your 'inner world' by taking courses in self-development. Perhaps there are enjoyable hobbies you've been putting off for later.

Taking part in these activities right now is part of balanced living. Moving towards meaningful goals is great, but we must also practice enjoying the present. This attitude can also be a big boost in the realm of stress management.

Stress And Culture

Some personality traits are very beneficial and help us to either handle the difficult situations that we face in life, or to stay relaxed as our life unfolds. Other traits are stress-inducing and can even cause us to create 'mountains out of molehills.'

We are generally all equipped with a combination of each of these traits: resilient personality traits that we have developed through overcoming challenges, personality traits that help us to stay relaxed and present, and other personality traits that push us towards distress. Of course, these traits can be changed with time.

All of us have unique personality traits which are a combination of resilient, relaxing, and stress-inducing. The larger groups we are apart of also have their own personalities formed by the unique mindsets and values of the people in these groups. We can call this a **collective personality**.

Each group, which is basically just two or more people, has its own collective personality. Towns, cities, and villages are all unique in this regard. You can get a sense of what the personality in an area is like when you visit these places. Even just two people coming together in a marriage has its own collective personality. Some of these personalities you may enjoy being around, and others, not so much.

In the Midwest, where I grew up, people are often known for being slower moving and friendlier than people living in a big city like New York or Boston. People living in Colorado have become known for living with a relaxed and open-minded attitude. The culture in Southern California is often considered by many to be more glamorous and superficial.

It's difficult to deny the influence that culture and a collective personality can have on us as individuals. You may have known someone who moved from a city to a small town and became more relaxed and slow moving. You may have also known somebody who moved from a small town to a big city and became transformed by the fast pace of city life.

Culture includes the morals, values, arts, and accepted ways of being of the people in a particular area. I would define **collective personality** as the consistent attitude, actions, and personality traits of people in that given area. Obviously, culture and collective personality are very similar and influence each other.

None of us are immune to the influence that culture and a collective personality can have on us. How then, would you define the collective personality in the area where you are living? In many ways, the United States, where I live, has taken on many of the Type A personality qualities that I described previously. These include competitiveness, striving, and serious focus. Our culture often values these qualities above the more easy-going and laid back qualities of the Type B personality.

Certainly, there are many people of all personality types in this country, but there seems to be a strong push for people to take on more of an *unbalanced* Type A functioning when it comes to work and life. I believe that this has put great pressure on the people living in this country and is a big cause of our individual stresses and strains. I have even seen this attitude sneak into school systems and put intense pressure on the achievement of children as young as six.

Questions to Consider
1. How are your thoughts and actions influenced by the culture you are a part of?
2. Do the thoughts and attitudes of your family and friends cause you to feel more distressed, or more relaxed?
3. How are your thoughts and actions influenced by your more local community, such as your town or city?
4. How much stress do you want to have in *your* life?

In the book *Tuesdays With Morrie*, the old professor (Morrie) says, "If the culture doesn't fit, then don't buy it." We live in a culture whose values don't usually help us to live a balanced and healthy life.

We are often pushed to do things that we don't enjoy simply for the sake of acquiring more. In our heart of hearts we yearn to express qualities of generosity, giving, and caring- both to ourselves and to others. We also yearn to live life with more relaxation and expression of individual differences. If the larger culture we belong to doesn't support these yearnings, then we may have to make a radical choice on the individual level to break free from cultural norms and live based on our own values.

In every developed country of the world, there are different cultures and collective personalities. In Italy, for example, it is common for people to take a two-hour lunch break from work and to go home and and have a joyous meal with their families. The Italian's, like many European cultures, consider a full work week to consist of 30 hours rather than the 40-60 hour workweek that is seen in the United States. The Italians are known for taking many more vacation days than the Americans, having much better health, and living life with much less distress.

In Italy, the collective personality has become much more closely aligned with the Type B personality over the Type A personality. They have decided, as a collective, that it's more important for them to spend time with friends and family, and to feel relaxed, instead of working at a furious pace to acquire more 'stuff.'

A Collective Solution to Stress

If there were a small recommendation that I could make to our entire U.S. culture for better managing stress, it would be to slightly change the way that we define *success*. Success is currently equated with the gaining of money and resources. The 'American Dream' that we were brought up with is all about the pursuit of fame and fortune.

I think that money and resources are perfectly worthy goals, but what are they truly worth if a great deal of health and happiness is sacrificed in there pursuit? If we as a society began having a broader and more **holistic** view of success, then we may each be able to experience financial prosperity, peace of mind, healthy relationships, and good health into old age. We could define *success* as the total attainment of physical, mental, emotional, spiritual, and financial well-being. (Not just financial prosperity).

Children could be brought up with a different idea of what it means to be *successful.* They could be asked to really consider what success looks like to them, rather than having it be assumed.

If we changed our definition of success to a broader and more holistic view, people may be encouraged to take better care of themselves. Employers may be more encouraged to support employee health. This attitude may even spill-over and cause us to take better care of the natural environment which is our home.

"Passion is energy. Feel the energy of
focusing on what excites you."
~Oprah Winfrey

On Energy and Balance

According to Dr. James Wilson, who has consulted many people suffering from adrenal fatigue and burn-out, the number one complaint of people who are chronically stressed is tiredness and fatigue.

Chronic stress burns through our precious resources quickly, and leaves our bodies and minds needing rest in order to rebuild and restore. Every distress that the body experiences creates an imbalance that must be dealt with. These all take *energy* to correct. It's no wonder that if a person has many sources of distress in their lives, they will inevitably complain of tiredness and fatigue.

On the flip side, the better you get at reducing, eliminating, and managing the stressors in your life, the more energy you will have. Plain and simple.

When is the last time you saw a group of children playing? Children are known for having an abundance of energy that seems almost inexhaustible. When I've been with groups of people where there are adults and children all together, I've often heard the adults envying how much energy the children have. The adults miss having that same liveliness.

What separates adults and children, in this matter, is not that as we grow older our energy naturally withers away. The children simply have less distress to deal with than the adults.

An adult who lives in a state of balance will actually have an energy level that is equal to, if not greater, than that of a child. They will be able to do everything that a child can do but won't need as much sleep. As we grow into middle-age, our bodies and minds should become more capable, not less. I've even known many people of the 75+ age group who took good care of themselves, and as such, had an abundance of energy into their later years.

If you want to have more energy, then seek to balance your stress levels.

If you want to have a lot of energy, then balance your stress *plus* find meaningful projects that you are passionate about to engage in. The thrill of seeking to accomplish these projects will fuel you.

Part 3

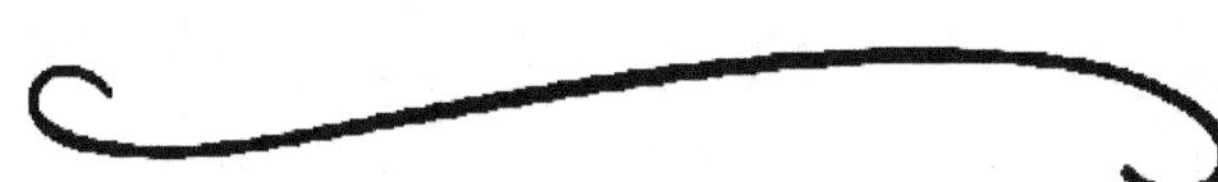

The Six Pillars of Living Life With More Energy and Less Stress

Your Stress Management Routine

We human beings are very capable of living a life that we enjoy. Living in a state of chronic stress can cause us to forget that fact.

Improved stress management will help us to bring our bodies and minds into a better state of balance, so that we can enjoy the pleasures and beauties of living life. There is likely no limit to just how balanced we can become.

Unfortunately for many, there are no pills or prescription medicines that make chronic stress go away. Medicine will not come into play until the wear and tear on the body or mind from too much distress has lead to an illness.

My life experience thus far has included many day-to-day stressors that I've had to learn to manage. I have also gone through about three periods of intense chronic stress, that forced me to adapt and evolve, so that I could regain a sense of peace. Once overcoming these challenges, there has always been new stressful experiences that I had to once again learn to adapt to. I'm sure that you've had plenty of your own stressful moments.

One thing that has improved for me over time, and which will improve for you as well, is that I've learned how to better handle stressful experiences as they arise. In this, I'm now more capable of bouncing back from pitfalls and handling difficult circumstances. I stay committed to practicing my favorite stress management techniques, and this has really allowed me to have more energy, mental clarity, and peace of mind.

Through conversations and research, I have come to realize that there are a collection of common practices and strategies that people can turn to in order to overcome distress and it's causes. I have selected six that appear to be very impactful and frequently turned to…

<u>The Six Pillars of Stress Management</u>
1. Triggering Relaxation
2. Doing What You Love
3. Joyful Movement
4. Social Support
5. The Art of Eating
6. Managing Time & Money

Improving your skill in just one or two of these areas can make a significant impact. It's often been seen that people have no real strategy in place for managing stress until they absolutely need to do so. It just isn't something that is taught to many people.

I've also noticed that many people already have decent strategies in place for managing stress, but aren't really conscious that they are doing so. Connecting with good friends, for example, can be a great strategy in times of distress, and people will often do so without even realizing it. Some people, as they age, become good at just 'brushing things off' and moving on from stressful experiences without concern. For others, that is easier said than done.

Some people already have decent stress management strategies in place, but then an event like a loss or a significant change occurs. This event, and the distress it causes, can overwhelm their stress management strategies sort of like a river breaking down a barrier. The individual is then forced to increase the measures that they take to reduce or eliminate emotional distress, so that they can feel healthy and at peace once again.

Whatever your **stress management routine** may encompass, pick some strategies that work well for you, and commit to doing them often. In today's world, it's good to have as many strategies and tools in place as possible.

Making Stress Management a Habit

If you can find people that will hold you accountable to practicing stress management techniques, that can be very helpful in adopting these new habits. **Accountability partners** will improve your chances of developing and sticking to *any* new habit. These are people close to you, who will help you to stay committed, and accountable, to your new habits and goals.

Here are a few more tips to help you adopt new and healthy stress management techniques into your day or week. They can also be used with other healthy habits that you may wish to adopt:

1. Schedule stress management strategies into your day. Scheduling time for important things, and then letting others know that you are busy during these times, will make relaxation and stress management easier to practice. You will want to 'block off' some time for this. That way, your new habits will be more honored and respected. This will be discussed further in pillar 6 on time management.

2. Give yourself rewards. According to Charles Duhigg, in his book *The Power of Habit*, the human brain pushes an individual to take part in routines for the reward that is provided in doing so. If you can give yourself a little snack or a treat after performing a new technique, this may make it easier to return to that technique and make it a habit. Providing yourself with a gift after a week or a month of adopting a new habit, may give that habit a more positive association in your mind. If your stress management practices lead to your feeling better, this may very well be enough reward and you won't need to provide any other goodies.

3. Pick stress management activities that you enjoy. Any healthier habit that you are adding to your life will be easier to adopt if you really enjoy it. For example, if you are someone that enjoys hiking in nature, then the hike itself will both balance stress levels and be self-rewarding. If the idea of getting dirty in a forest isn't your cup of tea, then maybe a nightly bath with candles and essential oils will be your new stress management practice.

4. Start small. One of the reasons that people try and fail when it comes to adopting new healthy habits is that they want to accomplish all of their goals right away. A new gym member, for example, may exercise like hell for a few days, and then when they realize that they haven't gotten into the shape that they hoped to be in all at once, they get discouraged and give up. This is an 'all or nothing' attitude. If you want to adopt a new stress management practice into your life, starting with just 15 minutes of deep breathing or walking each day can make a significant shift.

5. Be SMART. SMART stands for Specific, Measurable, Attainable, Relevant, and Time-based. A new habit that is based on these principles will be more successful than one which is missing any of these elements. A non-SMART goal may sound something like this, "I'm going to give guided visualizations a try." A SMART goal sounds like this, "I will meditate for 15 minutes every morning, for one week, using the words "peace and love" as a mantra. I will sit in my soft, comfy chair." The more specific, measurable, attainable, and time-based a goal becomes, the higher it's chances of accomplishment.

6. Get Creative. If you have to take a cab or a train home after work, the time that it takes to get there may be just what you need to practice some form of mental relaxation. A nice walk could be adopted after lunch at work. As a father, I've found all kinds of creative ways to include stress management into my daily life, along with work and family time.

Healthy vs. Unhealthy Coping Strategies

The techniques contained within my *Six Pillars of Living Life With More Energy and Less Stress* are health-enhancing ways of managing stress. This is because they really balance a person's body and mind, without negative side-effects. In the long run, they can help an individual to really be happier and healthier. The techniques in the *six pillars* will prepare you to better deal with stress as it arises.

Many coping strategies that people adopt for handling stress are actually health-diminishing in the long run. Several addictions, for example, are a person's way of simply avoiding the stress that they are experiencing. There are both substance-based addictions, and behavioral addictions, such as excessive shopping, working, and TV binging. Even a healthy habit can become an addiction if not practiced in moderation. You will know if you have an **addiction** because there will be negative consequences associated with that behavior.

Healthy stress management techniques, on the other hand, can actually help an individual to overcome or replace an addictive behavior. This is because many addictive behaviors are simply unhealthy ways of coping with distress. Relieve the distress, and the behavior may become uninteresting.

The Last Element of Recovery: Time

It's valuable to point out that if you are feeling chronically stressed or burnt-out, it will take some time to recover. No *one* technique will lift you from the discomfort of chronic stress in a single day.

The road back to recover your lost energy will also come with some setbacks. Healing is not linear. If you stick to your stress management practices, then the energy that you lost, <u>will</u> eventually return.

If you are one of the few people who has little to no distress in your life, that's great! In that case, you can still make a habit of practicing stress management techniques. That way, you are even more prepared to deal with distress as it arises.

You can also use several stress-balancing techniques, such as proper exercise and meditation, to move into higher modes of functioning. That way, you will be more capable of happiness, financial prosperity, and career success. Stress management techniques can honestly give you a real advantage in the workplace. A person in the home or office with a calm and peaceful presence can positively influence others and be very successful.

The most important factor in better managing stress will be your commitment. If you are ardently committed to living life with more energy and less stress, it is unlikely that you will fail.

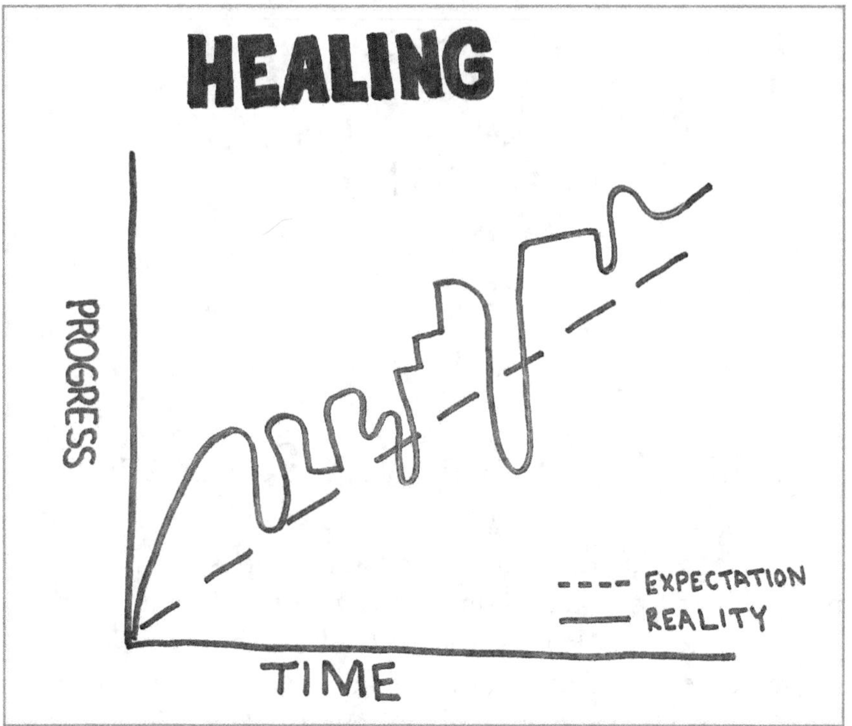
HEALING
PROGRESS
EXPECTATION
REALITY
TIME

20

Pillar 1 ~ Triggering Relaxation

Triggering the body's relaxation response is crucial to managing stress. That's honestly why it's listed as the first pillar. As stated in Part 2, when the relaxation response is triggered heart and breath rate will decrease, the body will have improved digestive capability, and thinking will be clearer. It is much easier for a relaxed person to be happy than a distressed person. Truly relaxing is not just a feeling or a cute phrase, relaxation has a powerful restorative effect on the body and mind of an individual.

Triggering relaxation can be done in many different ways. It is also something that can be learned to do and improved with practice.

Just as we all have unique personalities and abilities to handle stress, we can all find different ways to *relax*. Relaxation is imperative for good health and longevity. In a relaxed state, the body and mind have the greatest opportunities to repair and rebuild. Some relaxation techniques can even be more healing than sleep!

A **relaxation technique** is any activity we routinely take part in that triggers the relaxation response of the body. Relaxation techniques are many and varied. Some of them involve movement, some of them work with the breath, and others work with the mind. Some techniques, such as nature walking, are more active, and others, like sound bathing, are more passive. You likely have at least one thing in your life that you already engage in which helps you to relax in a health-promoting way.

A Note on Television and Internet Use

The average American watches television and uses the internet for a combined three to four hours daily. While browsing the internet and watching TV are activities that are often enjoyed, or simply taken part in, they are not generally able to be considered *relaxation techniques*. This is because they don't often trigger the bodies actual relaxation response. Only a few TV programs can be considered an exception.

Watching the national news, for example, is more likely to lead someone to feeling stressed and fearful, as opposed to relaxed. Enjoying a sports game may trigger eustress if your team does well, but if your team performs poorly, this can actually be very stressful. If an individual has a distressing day at work, and then comes home to simply watch distressing TV programming, this will only add to their distress load.

If you want to use television or internet to truly relax, you will have to be **very** selective of your programming. Otherwise, more productive relaxation techniques should be favored.

In Part 1 of this book on *Identifying Your Stressors* it was mentioned that there are three different ways to relieve or reduce a stressor:
1. Eliminate it from your life completely.
2. Better adapt to it.
3. Practice techniques to relieve the distress outside of it (Coping or Relaxing).

Say, for example, you are a girl named Judith, and you are having relationship difficulties with your boyfriend, Micky. These relationship difficulties are causing you to feel uncomfortable, upset, and giving you anxiety. The three options that you have to deal with this stressor are: 1. Practicing relaxation or coping methods to handle the distress, 2. Better adapting to the distress (which could involve going to couples counseling to improve communication), or 3. You could leave the relationship. If instead, you 'stuff down' the distress you are feeling and do nothing about it, you will be missing an opportunity for growth and simply suffering.

Rather than simply suffering, a more proactive approach should be taken. At certain times, we may have to take very proactive measures, which could indeed mean eliminating a stressor from our lives entirely. For Judith, this could mean ending her relationship with Micky. For another person, that may mean quitting a distressing job to go off on their own.

Keep in mind, that sometimes, the elimination of one stressor may simultaneously create other stress or stressors. If Judith were to end her relationship with Micky, for example, she may feel grief over the ending of the relationship.

At certain times, eliminating a stressor simply isn't possible.

Say, for example, a beloved friend has left town and it's caused you to feel lonely in their absence. You miss them and aren't sure if you will see them again. This loneliness is causing you some emotional distress. Or say, for example, you have some debt that is constantly weighing on you, and you find yourself being distressed about it. These two scenarios are examples of times where it's simply not possible to eliminate stressors. What *is* possible, is finding ways to both relax and to better cope with the stressor.

Relaxation techniques and **coping strategies** are not the same thing. Relaxation techniques trigger the body's relaxation response and can make us more relaxed individuals in the face of stressors. Coping strategies, on the other hand, give us the ability to either release or 'vent off' discomfort and distress.

Let's discuss the concept of coping further… Coping strategies help us as individuals to relieve or to release uncomfortable emotions, or physical pains, that have come about as a result of some stressor(s). A physical coping strategy could involve rubbing pain-relieving gel on an injured joint or muscle. The injury will still need to heal, but the pain relief will be appreciated.

Coping with mental/emotional distress is like rubbing pain relief on our emotions but is a bit more involved. Coping strategies to handle mental/emotional distress are meant to take the distress we are already feeling and express it in a way that causes us to feel some relief. Here are some *healthy* coping strategies for relieving mental/emotional distress:

<u>Coping Strategies</u>
- Writing out thoughts/feelings in a journal
- Expressing emotions through music and dance
- Yelling into a pillow
- Vigorous exercise
- Venting to a friend or receiving counseling
- Looking at a situation in a different way (Cognitive Reframing)

- Self-Pleasuring
- Crying or Laughter
- Caring for another living thing: person, animal, or plant
- Receiving a massage

Coping strategies are a great way to relieve distress and should definitely be applied when needed. Crying, for example, is simply the body's way of relieving distress that comes in the form of sadness, upset, or even anger. Many people have forgotten how to cry because it was discouraged when they were younger. If crying can be re-learned, it will serve as an excellent coping strategy.

Practicing relaxation at home can dump all the stress out of our bodies after a long day. Certain techniques, like deep breathing, can also be practiced at the moment distress is noticed to make us feel more relaxed.

Practicing relaxation can have cumulative benefits that spill-out into our days and make us more relaxed people in general. A person who practices yoga and mindfulness every morning, for example, may notice that things which used to be distressing for themselves, no longer cause distress. The body and mind are very habitual, and if you make the practice of relaxation a habit, then you are more likely to operate in a relaxed capacity. The opposite is also true.

Turning Attention Within

Many of the relaxation methods we will cover involve turning our attention from the 'outer world' back to the 'inner world' of thoughts, feelings, and sensations. Turning our attention from what's going on around us back to what's happening inside of our bodies, naturally helps our bodies move towards balance and homeostasis.

The outer world of work, people, and material objects will constantly be begging for our attention. For that reason, we will have to be committed to turning our attention inwards as an act of self-healing and self-compassion.

Relaxation Methods

We will go into several methods for triggering relaxation. Practice makes progress, so triggering relaxation, with any method(s), is a skill that will improve with practice. It's also good to note that there are cumulative benefits to practicing relaxation. The more you relax, the more benefits you will receive in the long run. If there are methods that you already use to trigger relaxation that are not on this list, keep practicing them. Here is an overview of the methods:
1. Deep 4-4 Breathing
2. Guided Visualization
3. Mantra Meditation
4. Thankfulness Prayers
5. Music Bathing
6. Relaxed Stretching
7. Nature Walking/Bathing
8. Hot Water Baths

Preparing to Relax

Practicing a relaxation technique can be done as a daily routine, or anytime that we notice we have some extra time to relax and unwind. If we find ourselves in the grip of the stress response, then it can be very helpful to practice relaxation as an emergency measure to regain our composure.

Practicing a relaxation technique in the same place and at the same time, every single day, can be beneficial because our mind and body will get into the habit of triggering relaxation routinely. If you want to experiment with relaxation techniques, feel free to approach it with a *playful* attitude. In a lot of ways, seriousness is a stress-prone attitude, whereas playfulness and curiosity lead to relaxation.

Once you have scheduled a place and time where you would like to relax, feel free to 'set the mood'. Light a candle, wear loose clothing if possible, and make sure that the area you are practicing in has as few distractions as possible. Obviously, if your relaxation time has come more spontaneously, then just do the best you can with what you've got, wherever you are. A car seat can even make a relaxation space when necessary.

Outdoors can be a great place to sit and relax as long as the weather conditions are favorable and there aren't too many bugs.

Body Positioning

A favorable physical position should be chosen for your relaxation session. The most favorable position could entail walking, sitting on a chair, sitting cross-legged, or lying flat on the floor. This will depend on the relaxation technique one has chosen. Whichever position *is* chosen, it should minimize any and all discomforts as much as possible. Pain and discomfort are not conducive to relaxation.

Sitting cross-legged is a position that has long been practiced for relaxation techniques such as deep breathing and meditation. If you enjoy sitting cross-legged and find it comfortable, then this can be a great position. If not, then ditch it. You can go into a very deep state of relaxation sitting in a chair, and you won't have to deal with any leg soreness that sitting cross-legged can lead to.

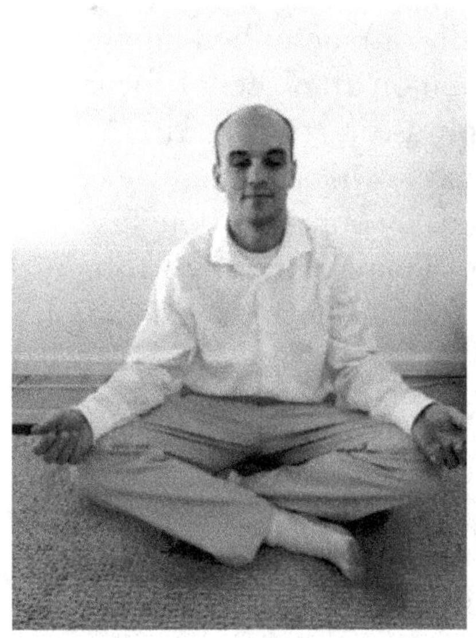

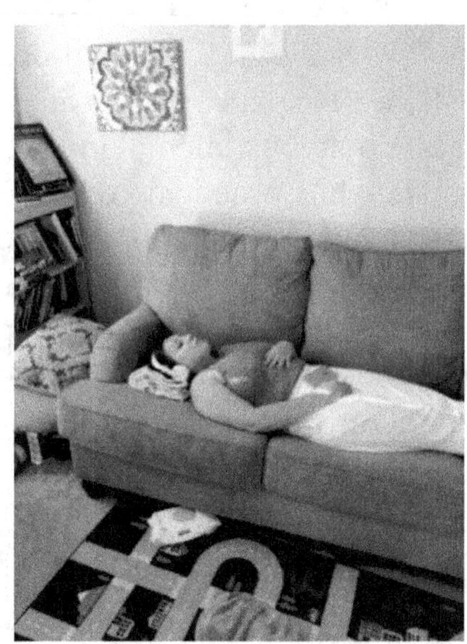

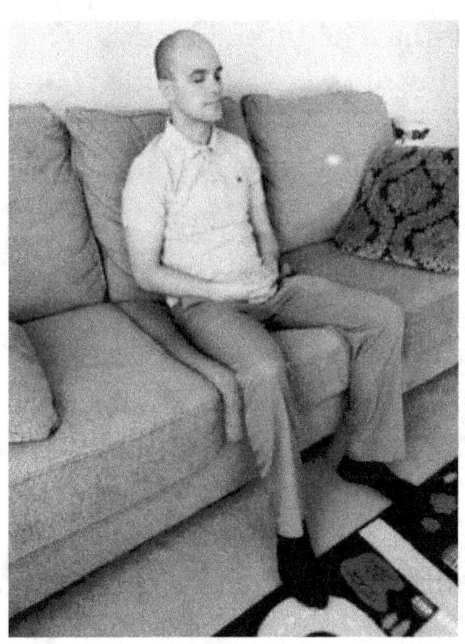

These images depict excellent relaxation postures. The most favorable posture will depend on the relaxation technique chosen.

Allowing Thoughts, Gentle Favoring

Several of the methods that are described (methods 1-5) involve placing one's attention on an object of focus. This could be a mental image, phrase, or the breath. At times, while practicing relaxation, it is possible that we can get distracted from the object of focus by our own thoughts, mental images, or daydreaming. There is nothing wrong with this. It is natural and to be expected. The art of relaxation in methods 1-5 involves five principles:

1. Getting Comfortable
2. Intending To Relax
3. Releasing Tension
4. Gently Favoring the Object of Focus
5. Allowing Thoughts, Feelings, and Images to Arise Without Resistance

So if thoughts, feelings, and images do arise, simply let them be. There is a good chance that the thoughts and feelings, which do arise, are coming about as a way for your body and mind to process either some excitement or stress. At times, these thoughts and images can even be 'dark' or angry. Allowing these things to be as they are and allowing your mind to process them, will be a big help in the long run.

If you find that you have some persistent thoughts about things that need to be done, then you can keep a notebook nearby while you relax, and write these thoughts down. This way, you won't have to worry about forgetting your task, and you can return to your notes later.

Relaxation can be considered an art form, and just like any art form, a person will become more skilled with practice.

Method 1~ Deep 4-4 Breathing

Deep and rhythmic breathing is a very valuable stress management skill to learn because it can be practiced almost anytime, anywhere. It can also be very effective for triggering relaxation.

When the body goes into either anxiety or panic from distress, breathing will normally become shallow and rapid. People scurrying about their day in the 'fight or flight' mode are constantly breathing this way.

Breathing deeper into the lungs, and breathing rhythmically, can intercept the bodies stress response and cause a person to feel relaxed and experience some clarity.

<u>Deep 4-4 Breathing Technique</u>:
1. Sit comfortably in a chair or lay on a comfortable surface.
2. Straighten your spine and allow your body to relax.
3. Breathe into the deepest part of your lungs as you slowly count in your head 1, 2, 3,4. Exhale to the slow count of 1, 2, 3, 4. Breathe into the deepest part of your lungs 1, 2, 3, 4. Exhale 1, 2, 3, 4.
4. And that's it. If you are practicing at home do this for 10 - 15 minutes.

The more you practice your skill with this deep, 4-4 rhythmic breathing, the more effective it can become as a relaxation technique.

You can practice deep 4-4 breathing while at a desk, while standing, or even while driving to work. If you notice yourself feeling routinely distressed during your commute to work, give this breathing technique a good attempt as an intervention. You can do this by minimizing all distractions in the car (such as turning off the radio) and practice deep 4-4 breathing as you drive. You may get to work feeling much calmer and more mentally and emotionally prepared.

Deep 4-4 breathing can also be combined with other methods such as relaxed stretching and music bathing.

Method 2 ~ Guided Visualization

Visualization is a technique that can be used for several different purposes. There are professional athletes who use visualization to imagine themselves winning a major sports competition. I have heard of other people using visualization to imagine themselves moving on after the ending of a relationship.

Here we will use visualization *to relax.*

Relaxing visualization involves using the imagination to visualize a beautiful nature scene or another safe place. This will send a message to the body that everything is well, and it's fine to relax, let go, and heal.

Any time that a person uses their imagination to picture themselves in trouble or danger, the imagination is being used to trigger the stress response. Anyone who has ever used the imagination in this way, knows that the physiological response to these images or thoughts can be very powerful.

The physiological response of using your imagination to visualize safety and comfort can also be very powerful.

For this technique we will use the help of technology such as a computer, mp3 player, or cell phone. If a cell phone is used, make sure that it is switched to airplane mode.

Guided Visualization Technique:
1. Get into a comfortable position. Make sure that you are free from distractions.
2. Put on headphones connected to an mp3 player, phone, or laptop.
3. Go on the website YouTube.com and search the phrase 'Relax For A While.' You will get several search results

from the YouTube channel Relax For A While. You can pick one of the guided nature visualizations to listen to in order to relax and unwind. Alternatively, you can find your own visualization to enjoy.

4.   After the visualization is over, it can be wise to take a couple of minutes to lay calmly with your eyes closed before re-entering the world.

Method 3 ~ Mantra Meditation

Using a short phrase or 'mantra' repeated over and over in the mind is one of the oldest relaxation techniques on Earth. It is actually one of my favorite ways to relax. I enjoy using the phrase "Be Still and Know That I Am God" which comes from the Bible (Psalms 46:10).

If you are concerned that practicing meditation either goes against your spiritual beliefs or doesn't conform to your world-view, then feel free to skip this section.

On the other hand, I would encourage anyone who hasn't meditated before, to give it a try, and approach it with an open mind. Mediation is simply a way to relax and to tune into the potential that a balanced mind and body can afford an individual.

If you do have a concern about meditation and your religious affiliation, but you would still like to meditate, then I would encourage you to adapt this technique to *your* religious world-view. In terms of the 'mantra,' this could involve choosing a phrase that is sacred within your religious group.

If you do not have a sacred phrase that you want to repeat, then simply use the phrase 'I Love Life,' 'Peace and Kindness,' or another emotionally positive sequence of words. You can also choose to recite a sound that is void of meaning such as 'Shuh-Ream.' Reciting sounds that don't have a meaning can actually be valuable, because your mind will not get attached to the meaning of the words.

<u>Mantra Meditation Technique</u>:
1. For this technique, it is encouraged that you sit up straight in a chair or sit cross-legged. Lying down is not suggested in this case because it is very conducive to sleeping. So get in a comfortable sitting position.
2. Choose a word or a phrase that you can recite over and over and that you enjoy repeating.
3. Gently recite that word or phrase over and over in your mind, not worrying about the cadence, pace, or speed of the recitation.
4. When your focus becomes distracted with thoughts, allow the thoughts to be present, but gently bring your attention back to the mantra.
5. Practice this technique for twenty minutes. The morning is best.
6. When finished, lie on the floor for a few minutes, or sit with eyes open, before returning to activity.

Mantra Mediation can be an excellent way to relax and to allow the mind to process any uncomfortable emotions, worries, or fears. If you feel very tired at any time during the practice, feel free to stop the mantra, lay down, and relax. If you do fall asleep, this can be very rejuvenating sleep, because you will be going into it in a very relaxed state. If you want to learn more on this technique, I would suggest a book called *Deep Meditation* by Yogani.

Method 4 ~ Thankfulness Prayers

Saying prayers of thankfulness is a practice for cultivating positive emotions. The prayers of thankfulness can be directed towards God or a higher power, if one wishes. If one does not have a belief in a higher power, this technique can still be practiced. You can choose whether you want to say "thank you God for __" or simply, "thank you for ___ occurring/being in my life."

Whether or not you believe in a higher power, this technique can be very powerful and **VERY** relaxing. Contemplating what we are thankful for and then saying *thank you* for these people, events, conditions, or objects will produce positive thoughts. Positive thoughts will then trigger positive emotions, leading to a flood of feel-good hormones dispersed throughout the body, as well as feelings of relaxation.

For this technique, it's great to have a string of prayer beads or a rosary to help us keep count of our prayers. If you move one bead further on the string each time you say a prayer, intending to get around the whole string, then this will give you a worthy goal to aim for. A rosary usually has 59 beads on it. If you have a string of Indian mala beads, this will give you 108 prayers.

If you don't have one of these available, then you can just count in your head "1,2,3, etc." No matter how you keep count, the intention we will set is to reach a goal of at least 100 thankfulness prayers during a session. This could involve two rotations around a string of rosary beads, for example.

<u>Thankfulness Prayer Technique</u>:
1. Sit comfortably in a chair or on a seat.
2. Contemplate everything that improves the condition of your life in any way. Contemplate this for a minute or two.
3. Hold the first prayer bead in your fingers or gently say "1." Then, state what you are thankful for, whether it be a person, event, circumstance, or object- anything that improves your life.
4. Move to the next bead, or gently say "2," and then again, say what you are thankful for.
5. Continue saying prayers of thanks until you reach at least 100. If using a rosary, this will mean going around the string twice.

Method 5 ~ Music Bathing

Music bathing simply refers to listening to music in a very calm and intentional fashion. You let your body lie still while allowing the sounds of the music to just 'wash over' you. Music bathing is most effective when approached with the attitude to really lie still and surrender your mind, body, and awareness to the sounds of the music.

Obviously, for this technique, music selection will be paramount. Not all music will be conducive to producing relaxation within the body. Most heavy metal, pop, and rap music, for example, is more likely to trigger either liveliness or alertness, as opposed to feelings of deep relaxation. Music that is instrumental and without words or lyrics will be the best choice for relaxing. Music with lyrics that is acoustic could also be used, if you know for sure that it triggers relaxation within you. I have witnessed my Father relaxing to the gentle acoustics and singing of Simon and Garfunkel, for example.

If you are not aware of music that you can use to relax with at this moment, then experiment with the selections below. These artists create music specifically for the sake of relaxation. You can look up these albums either for free on YouTube or purchase them from a store like iTunes. (Purchasing the music is preferable as it will be played without interruption from advertisements.)

Albums for Relaxation
- *A New Kind of Love* by Robin Spielberg
- *Intervention* by Helen Jane Long
- *Dolphin Dreams* by Dan Gibson
- *Imagination's Light* by Kevin Kern
- *New Life* by Paul Cardall

<u>Music Bathing Relaxation Technique</u>:
1.   Pick a selection of music that you know you can relax to.
2.   Lie in a comfortable position and play your music.
3.   Allow your body to really relax in place and listen to the music with a gentle focus. Notice each note as the sound moves through your body.
4.   When you notice that you are distracted from the listening of music by thoughts or images, simply *gently favor* the music with your focus.
5.   This technique can be done for any length of time. 30 to 60 minutes is ideal.

Method 6 ~ Relaxed Stretching

Relaxed Stretching can be done to both trigger relaxation and promote mind-body integration. The most popular form of relaxed stretching performed in the United States is very likely Yoga Asanas. As Yoga has swept across the country, it has proven it's stress-relieving potential to both it's fanatics and novice participants alike.

Many studies have now been done on the practice of Yoga Asanas, revealing the effectiveness that this system can have on both balancing cortisol levels and relieving the symptoms of distress.

As Yoga has become popular, there have become many types of Yoga classes offered. If you want to practice Yoga for stress relief, aim specifically for classes that promote mind-body integration. My suggestion to you, if you'd like to practice Yoga Asanas for stress relief, is to either go to a Sivanada Yoga class or see if you can find a good Yin Yoga class in your area. Several good teachers in other disciplines also stay in touch with the original mind-body integration aspects of Yoga.

The art of *relaxed stretching* is a way to practice either yoga asanas or simple stretches with the intention, and technique required, to really relax and let go. If you have either a Yoga video or remember some stretches you've done in the past, then relaxed stretching can easily be practiced at home.

The art of relaxed stretching involves not pushing oneself too far during a stretch, really focusing on the stretching sensation, breathing into the stretch, and not feeling rushed. If done correctly, stretching the muscles can lead to a limber body, a calm mind, and a refreshed feeling.

<u>Relaxed Stretching Technique</u>:
1. Sit comfortably on the floor for a moment.
2. Adopt the stretching posture you wish to practice.
3. Slowly begin the stretching of the muscles for the chosen posture. Go until you feel a gentle stretch, but not to the point of strong discomfort.
4. Put your awareness on the stretching sensation, and practice the Deep 4-4 Breathing technique as you do so. Imagine the breath going into the area of stretching.
5. Hold each posture for approximately 60 seconds before moving on to the next. Gently come out of the stretch when ready.
6. When all stretches that you wanted to accomplish are completed, lay on the floor and practice 4-4 Breathing for at least 3 minutes.
7. Enjoy the rest of your day.

Method 7 ~ Nature Walking/Bathing

"To the attentive eye, each moment of the year has its own
beauty, and in the same field, it beholds, every hour, a picture
which was never seen before, and which
shall never be seen again."
~Ralph Waldo Emerson, Nature

Leaving behind a busy town or city to go out into the
natural world and relax (termed 'nature bathing' or 'forest
bathing') can be rejuvenating and relaxing for body, mind,
and spirit. For thousands of years, people have gone out into
the natural world to take a break from the challenges of life
and to gain a broader perspective on what their life is about.
You can do this too.

There are several known reasons why nature bathing
can be good for our mental/emotional health and why it
triggers relaxation within the body and mind. Here are a few:
- The natural world often moves at a slower and more
  synchronized pace than the human world of cars, trains,
  and electronic devices. When 'bathing' in nature our minds
  and bodies will begin to synchronize with this slower pace.
- The natural world is rich with sensations from sights,
  sounds, and (mostly) delightful smells. Being in this field of
  sensation helps us to reconnect with our own bodies and
  sensory organs.
- Everything that runs on energy, including all living beings
  and electronics, emits a measurable electromagnetic
  frequency. It's been measured that every natural
  environment, including mountain forests, meadows, and the
  natural areas surrounding bodies of water, all resonate at an
  electromagnetic frequency of 7.8 hZ. This is known as the
  Schumann Resonance. This 7.8 hZ frequency has also
  come to be known as the 'frequency of homeostasis,'

because when our bodies are subjected to this frequency they naturally move towards greater balance (homeostasis). Going out into the natural world will influence our own electromagnetic fields to harmonize with the Schumann Resonance emitted by all plants and trees.

Excellent areas for the practice of nature bathing include lakes, oceans, forests, and meadows. Parks can even be helpful if that is the most accessible area you have. In Albuquerque, where I live, we are fortunate to have some very nice parks and a nature preserve that stretches the whole length of the Rio Grande River going through the city. If you have an area that you know would be good for nature bathing, you can take advantage of this spot for stress management and mental sanity.

To nature bath, it is ideal to slowly walk in a natural area, occasionally sit, and 'take in the sights.' There are even guide services that have successful businesses leading people on nature bathing experiences.

<u>The Nature Bathing Technique</u>:
1. Pick a natural area that you know will be good for nature bathing.
2. Make sure to dress properly for the occasion and wear a natural bug spray, if there is a need for it.
3. Go out into the nature area and leave your cell phone on airplane mode. We are trying to escape the human world- not bring it with us.
4. Engage the senses. As you move through the natural world, pay close attention to the sights, sounds, and smells around you. Feel free to touch some bark, sand, or leaves. It will also be good to sit and 'soak things in' occasionally.
5. When you notice your mind drifting off, bring your *gentle focus* back to the natural scenery that surrounds you.

6. Practice nature bathing for at least 30 minutes at a time, whenever you feel called to do so, or when you are caught up in the 'fight or flight' mode.

The natural world can be a great place for balancing the human mind and body. You may wish to write a journal entry on your experiences. You can also couple nature bathing with other techniques, such as mantra meditation, if there is a minimum amount of distractions.

Method 8 ~ Hot Water Baths

In the state of New Mexico, there are several hot-spring spas that people travel from far and wide to visit. *Ten Thousand Waves* in Santa Fe, New Mexico is one such establishment. They heat fresh spring water straight from the mountain to a comfortable 101 to 103 degrees Fahrenheit. People then soak in this hot mineral water, so that they can relax their muscles and joints and to trigger a deep state of relaxation and serenity. *Ten Thousand Waves* also features a meditation room where people are free to lay back, relax, and *just be.* I promise that I have no affiliation with them. I just like their 'vibe,' and I enjoy going there to relax, myself.

Taking a hot water bath is a luxury that our hunter-gatherer ancestors would have likely never even dreamed of. Taking a hot mineral bath can relieve joint and muscle pain and be very good for triggering relaxation. Likely, taking a hot bath is a short-cut to relaxation, because it mimics how we as unborn babies would have felt in the womb of our mothers.

In the womb, we were simply submerged in warm water, with all of our needs met, and not a care in the world. Visiting a hot spring bathhouse, relaxing in what's called a 'float tank,' or simply taking a hot bath at home, can all trigger the relaxation response by reminding us of how we felt in our mother's womb.

My wife seems to have mastered the art of turning a bathroom and a bath tub into a temple for peace and relaxation. This hot water bath technique is something that I have not mastered myself, just yet, but I have formulated the technique based on what I've observed.

I have also noticed that in several popular movies and T.V. shows the main female character will turn to a hot bath to trigger relaxation and to do some contemplation. Women in general, it would seem, are more sensitive to their bodies, emotions, and feelings than most men. For this reason, women are also good at using the power of their senses to trigger relaxation. No matter what your gender, this technique can be effective:

<u>Hot Water Bath Technique</u>:
1. Find a bathroom with a bathtub.
2. Light a couple of candles in this bathroom.
3. Play some relaxing music.
4. Turn off all other lights.
5. Take a hot bath and relax.

This hot water bath technique can also be aided by listening to some gentle music and following the *music bathing* instructions.

Other Techniques

If you aren't able to find at least one way to relax in today's world, you may very well be headed for chronic stress. Therefore, for health and sanity, it is imperative to find ways to relax and to then practice these techniques ritually.

The methods listed thus far do not encompass all possible relaxation techniques; this list is simply meant to give a person suggestions and inspiration. If you already have a relaxation technique that you practice, continue with that technique for as long as it feels good to do so.

There are several other potentially excellent techniques that one can practice. Here are some more methods that are proven either scientifically or subjectively to produce feelings of relaxation:
- Reading
- Writing
- Needle Arts
- Receiving a Massage
- Tai Chi
- Gardening
- Drinking Wine or Spirits in Moderation
- Making Woodwork
- Painting

Physical Discomforts

While relaxation techniques are overall enjoyable, it *is* possible to feel some discomfort as a symptom of relaxation. The physical discomforts that one may experience as a result of relaxation could be from: improper body positioning, trying too hard to relax, or from chemical re-balancing.

An example of trying too hard to relax could be focusing on a mantra so intensely, or seriously, that you end up giving yourself a headache. If this is experienced, simply discontinue relaxing for a while and lighten up.

It is also possible to experience some physical or emotional discomfort as a result of something called **chemical re-balancing**. This could look like a person really enjoying a relaxation technique while it is taking place, but then afterward feeling extremely tired or fatigued, or having the pain from an old injury flare-up. These things are not super common for the novice practitioner of relaxation to experience, but can happen. They come about as a result of the body of a person getting used to functioning in a very different capacity.

If a person is very accustomed to being 'on the go' and always in a rush, then relaxation will cultivate a very different functioning of mind and body for this person. This different functioning then creates a different hormonal and chemical environment within the body. This can potentially lead to the body wanting to heal an old injury, re-balancing itself, or desiring to rest. <u>If a person feels tired while practicing a relaxation technique, the best thing to do is to lie down and rest</u>. An alarm can be set if there is a concern about falling asleep.

While relaxation is generally pain free, some discomforts can occur. The best way to navigate most of these discomforts is to scale back on relaxing for awhile, and to rest.

Emotional Discomforts

I have seen many times in myself and others, where we will practice a relaxation technique, feel great during, but then feel some anger or sadness afterward. "What's going on here, we ask?"

While practicing relaxation, the body and mind may use this opportunity of slowing down to heal some unresolved 'emotional baggage.' If you practice relaxation and then afterward are feeling emotional, this is what is occurring.

Basically, every one of us is going through life with some unresolved emotional clutter. This could be from a harsh event we experienced in childhood, an unresolved breakup, the loss of someone in our lives that still troubles us… There are many times in life that we have neither the time nor resources to fully resolve a troubling emotional experience.

Practicing relaxation can, at times, awaken these emotions so that we can effectively process what's been tucked away. In the long run, this will help us to heal these emotions so that we no longer have to carry them around inside of us.

Many people go through their lives constantly running from their emotions. Practicing relaxation techniques can actually take a bit of courage, because it will put us more deeply in touch with our 'internal worlds' of thoughts, feelings, and emotions. If you have the courage to both make the time to relax and are willing to face your unresolved emotions, you will feel much better in the long run.

My suggestion to you, if you are feeling some emotional discomfort after a relaxation technique, is to simply lie down and rest for a while. After some rest, it can then be good to practice a coping technique to express the pent-up emotion. This could involve doing some journaling, light exercise, or playing an instrument if you have the ability.

Higher Power

Occasionally, practicing a relaxation technique can lead a person to feeling like they have come in communion with either their **soul** or a **higher power**. This does not always happen for people, but it certainly is wonderful to hear of someone having an amazing experience like this, when it does occur. Experiences like these are more likely to happen if one wishes, or intends, on having them.

Resistance to Practicing Relaxation

There are several reasons why an individual may not want to practice relaxation. Some of the biggest ones are: being afraid to confront our 'internal worlds,' feeling like relaxation is 'unproductive,' or feeling like it's not working.

We often have a mindset, as a society, that to be productive and to accomplish our goals, we need to be constantly doing something. We assume that when we are working and moving, this is the only time we are getting anywhere. While work and activity are obviously paramount to both our physical health and the achievement of our goals; relaxation can also be very productive.

Relaxation allows us to deeply rest and to prepare our bodies and minds, so that they are much more effective when we do act. Metaphorically, relaxation is a bit like sharpening a dull knife. Someone who prepares food in a restaurant can work all day with a dull knife and still accomplish some things, but they will work much faster and more efficiently if their knives are sharp while preparing the fruits and vegetables. When we practice relaxation techniques, we are "sharpening" our minds and bodies, so that they can work efficiently.

Relaxing deeply can also lead to the manifestation of mental insights and breakthroughs that we may not have otherwise had. Sometimes a mental breakthrough can be applied to our life, work, or relationships to make everything run more smoothly. In this way, insights and breakthroughs can make life easier and more enjoyable.

Both a good night's rest and relaxation have been known to allow solutions to challenges, and creative breakthroughs, to rise from our sub-conscious minds into our conscious awareness.

Optimal Balance

Even though practicing relaxation techniques is great for body, mind, and spirit; practicing them too often can still lead to an imbalance. For most people, just a small amount of intentional relaxation can make a big difference. Fifteen to twenty minutes of meditation every morning, for example, can really help a person to stay calm more often during the day. Thirty to sixty minutes of relaxation techniques a day can incur added benefits.

Beyond that, a balanced life will include relaxation <u>plus</u> all the other elements: activity, movement, work, leisure, etc.

Pillar 2 ~ Doing What You Love

As my parents taught me when I was a kid, "sometimes in life, we have to do things that we don't enjoy doing."

The reason that we do these things is that we see a value to them in the long run. I've never especially liked going to the dentist, for example, but I have found it to be a very valuable action to take for good oral health.

Although we all have to spend some time doing things we'd rather not be doing, distress arises when we spend most of our days doing things that don't ignite our 'inner flame.' Say, for example, you don't enjoy your job, plus you have a host of unenjoyable responsibilities to take care of outside of work. In this case, you will be experiencing what I would call **existential friction**. This existential friction occurs because in your mind you are doing what you feel you need to, but in your heart, you'd rather be living differently. This friction then creates a condition of mental/emotional distress within an individual.

On the other hand, doing things that you either really enjoy doing, or that you *love* to do, creates feelings of eustress, and is certainly favorable to doing things which you hate. Doing things that you love to do, or are interested in, leads to feelings of excitement and fulfillment. It makes life feel like it's worth living simply for its own enjoyment. Doing what you love to do helps you to understand your true desires for your life. In the doing of things that you love, the direction that you want your life to move in is more easily revealed, since people most often desire to spend time with people, and in places, that they love.

Un-enjoyable activities are usually done because of a sense of real or imagined responsibility. A life exclusively lived this way will create distress, bitterness, and discontent. If you notice that this is how your life is going, then it is time to reflect and contemplate on how you would rather live.

For reasons of financial or personal need, you may not be able to make drastic changes in your life at this moment. A person may not be able to end a job that no longer fits them, at this moment, for example. What you *can* do is to consider the things you really enjoy doing, what you would love to do more of, and then to start incorporating more of these activities into your life. This may include different hobbies, interests, or career possibilities that you've always wanted to explore.

The Hero's Journey

Author and Professor Joseph Campbell studied and wrote on a popular topic in literature called 'The Hero's Journey.' The Hero's Journey is a sequence of similar events that happen in almost all heroic fairy tales. The Hero's Journey involves the hero or heroine of the story first hearing a call to action. The hero will then (possibly with some reluctance) leave the safety and comfort of the familiar to face a great challenge or to go on an adventure. Once the hero or heroine is on this adventure, they will face great trials and setbacks. Their inner resources and spirit will be tested almost to their limit.

Eventually, the hero or heroine will accomplish the goal that they set out to accomplish- and along the way, they will likely receive some help from a guide or mentor. The hero or heroine, after completing their quest, will then venture home to where they started. They will have new abilities and a broader understanding of life. This similar sequence of events is seen in many of the beloved classics such as *The Lord of The Rings*, with Frodo Baggins being the hero; and the movie *Moana*.

Joseph Campbell said that the path to the hero's journey and the way to get through it, involves "following your bliss." He would often encourage his college students to do what they truly loved and to "follow their bliss." He said that for him, when he was doing what he really loved to do, "doors would mysteriously open." He also commented that if life is merely spent striving and struggling, "you can have some level of success, but what kind of a life is that?"

"I always tell my students, 'Follow Your Bliss.' Go where your Being, body, and soul wanna go. When you have that feeling, stay with it, and don't let anyone throw you off. If you do follow your bliss, you put yourself on a kind of track that has been there all the while waiting for you, and the life you ought to be living is the one you are living.

~Joseph Campbell

I'm not as old of a man as Joseph Campbell was when he taught others to follow their bliss, nor am I as wise. What I do know, is that when you fill your life with activities you enjoy doing, people are more likely to be attracted to you and give you opportunities. Your mind is happier. You will likely have much less distress and much more comfort.

'Following your bliss' and 'doing what you love' are almost synonymous. Another similar encouragement that I have been given is to "keep pursuing your interests." However you want to say it, there is an understanding amongst all wise people that if you want to enjoy your life, you need to do the things that naturally make you feel alive, excited, and inspired.

We are all the hero or heroine of our own story. To make our story a good one and to feel energized, we should all pursue our interests and do the things we love.

Meaning and Purpose

I believe that it is easiest to find meaning and purpose in life when we are helping other living beings in some way or another. When we feel like our actions are contributing to the well-being of people, animals, or the Earth as a whole, it is much easier to gain a sense of meaning or purpose.

If we can find a way to couple 'doing what we love' and being of assistance to others, then we are setting the stage for a life high on meaning and one low on existential friction. If our actions are only satisfying our sense of obligation to our responsibilities, then it is much harder to find a deeper meaning in what we are doing.

Starting Small

If you currently feel some existential friction in your life (or a lot), you don't need to start making big shifts immediately. Simply consider, what is it that I would rather be doing with my life, and what is one small step that I can take to get there? If there is a new career option that interests you, you could take on-line classes in your free time, for example.

If your life is full of responsibilities that you don't enjoy, maybe you could ask others for help with these duties.

If you aren't sure what you really enjoy doing in life, or what your interests are, then you could try out some of the relaxation techniques in Pillar 1 of this book. As stated previously, sometimes, when the body and mind are more relaxed, good ideas will percolate to the surface of our awareness.

Once you do find hobbies, activities, and work options that you really like doing, take small steps every day to fill your life with more enjoyment. It will be like rolling a small snowball down a hill that eventually builds up some momentum.

Making Bold Changes

At certain times in life, we do have to make bold choices to create a life we enjoy living. I have had times in my life where I've ended relationships, dropped out of college, packed up all my things and moved to a different state… Not all at once, but spread out over the years.

Once we feel strongly that a decision like this will lead to a more fulfilling existence for ourselves, then we have to act. In the long run, life will indeed get better.

Reframing

Reframing is a process of looking at the things in our lives in a different way. Reframing allows us to appreciate, or to see the value in, things which we may have been taking for granted- including ourselves.

Reframing is quite a bit different than "making bold changes," because rather than changing our circumstances, we choose to look at them more appreciatively.

If you feel strongly that you need to make a change, then by all means do so. In the long run, it will improve your health and sanity. But if you feel like a change isn't appropriate, then change how you look at the circumstances in your life to appreciate their value more.

If you currently have a challenge going on in your life that you must face, you could ask yourself, "what am I gaining from going through this circumstance?"

In your relationships, you could ask yourself, "how can I let this person know that I care about them, in order to improve the quality of the relationship?"

In a job setting, you can ask yourself, "what skills and qualities am I gaining from being in this environment?"

Reframing can help us to diffuse the tension that we may be feeling in a circumstance, and can allow us to improve the quality of our relationships- to work, family, and friends. Reframing can also help us to realize the positive aspects of what is going on in our lives.

'Doing What You Love' Questions to Ponder

1. What would you do with your life if you had all the money that you needed?
2. When your life feels most ideal, what is it that you are doing?
3. When you were younger, what subjects were you naturally drawn to?
4. What is it that you enjoy doing, simply for its own sake?

Pillar 3 ~ Joyful Movement

Just as it is important to allow the body and mind time for rest and recovery, it is also very important for optimal health and wellness, to move the body. Movement that is conducted for the sake of improving mental, emotional, and physical health is normally called 'physical activity' or 'exercise.'

I am choosing to name this pillar of stress management Joyful Movement, because I want to encourage the fact that physical activity can actually be very enjoyable, and that specific activities for stress management should be chosen based on the ways that one truly enjoys moving the body.

Many people, upon *just hearing* the word exercise will begin to grumble. They may remember times when they were forced to put on gym shorts during high school and run around in circles until they almost fainted. When people think of 'exercise' they may also think of models and body-builders; people who often exercise so much that they virtually live at the gym.

In naming this pillar of stress management Joyful Movement, I want to enhance the point that exercise is not only healthy; individuals can, and should, participate in physical activities that they really enjoy. Exercise is not about getting a gym membership and 'pumping iron' (unless this is your joy). Exercise, physical activity, or Joyful Movement can involve dancing, swimming, hiking, biking, love making, aerobics, or just walking.

When Joyful Movement is incorporated into a weekly routine, it gives an individual an improved chance of being healthy, living a long life, and enjoying life more. It enhances not only one's physical fitness and physical health, it is also great for mental and emotional well-being. Exercise is said by many specialists to be as good, or better, at relieving symptoms of depression than prescription drugs. It's also a great stress buster! Here are some of the top benefits of adding enjoyable movement to your routine:

1. Enhanced feelings of well-being.
2. Improved muscular strength and stamina.
3. Improved heart health.
4. Improved hormonal regulation (often leading to more positive emotions).
5. Release of beta-endorphins (responsible for 'runner's high').
6. Enhanced self-esteem.
7. Improved body composition.
8. Better quality sleep.
9. And of course, less distress.

If you would like to incorporate more exercise into your life for the myriad of health benefits that it provides, and going to the gym isn't your thing, no worries. Many good-quality exercises can be done at home, outdoors, in a dance studio, or in a pool.

Movement and Stress

The fascinating thing about physical activity and stress, is that physical activity raises adrenaline levels and places distress on the body in the short term, but then reduces mental/emotional stress and build a stronger body, in the long run. Shortly before a physical activity begins, the body will release some adrenaline to help you fuel your workout. Heart rate will rise, vision will focus-in, and the blood of the body will go to the muscles.

As physical activity is conducted, it then leads to the breakdown of muscles. After this initial breakdown, the body will then re-build the muscles, and also bones, stronger than they were before. For this process to be most effective, proper nutrients, rest, and water should be provided to the body.

Physical activity will also improve stress modulation in the long run. There are three stress-modulating benefits to physical activity:

- First, physical activity 'burns off' extra stress hormones like cortisol and adrenaline circulating inside of the body. Many people know this instinctively and will turn to physical activity in times of distress. Bouts of exercise lasting 30 minutes or longer will be excellent for 'burning off' the stress hormones that are released during daily struggles.
- Second, after exercise has ended, the level of stress hormones in the body will typically be lower than they were before the exercise routine began. This makes physical activity a very valid coping method in times of distress.
- Third, physical activity makes the body more resistant to distressing experiences in the long run. You see, the body gets more accustomed at processing adrenaline and cortisol as it does during physical activity, so when distress does arise, your body is better at returning to baseline faster.

Physical Activity for Stress Management

Almost any physical activity that is done safely will yield benefits for stress management. That being said, the best physical activity for managing stress is one that an individual truly enjoys taking part in. This can take the negativity people often associate with *exercise* and turn it into 'joyful movement.' For me, I love to swim, run a little, do some strength training, and play sports. An ideal exercise routine for me, involves doing each one of these activities once per week.

My wife loves to dance and run. She says that at times while she's running she, "feels like she's flying."

One very popular doctor in the U.S. is constantly touting the benefits of swimming as this exercise is both aerobic and maintains strong joints and muscles. He also loves the practice of it.

Whatever physical activity you enjoy doing is the one you should stick to. If you enjoy the physical activity you are taking part in, then you will most likely engage in it more often, you will incur less mental strain, and you can even produce positive stress (eustress) and go into the flow state.

Strength Training vs. Aerobic Activity

Generally speaking, there are two different modes of physical activity: strength training (which is anaerobic) being the first; and aerobic activity, such as running, brisk walking, and biking being the second. The second mode, aerobic activity (also called "cardio"), is better for relieving distress. This is because aerobic activities burn through the stress hormones faster.

That being said, strength training is a very valuable activity for keeping the body strong and toned throughout one's life span. The Physical Activity Guidelines for Americans is a book put out every 5 years by the U.S. Department of Health and Human Services. This book, which is authored by top experts in the field of fitness, recommends strength training at least twice per week for all adults. This could involve weight lifting for 2-4 "sets" twice per week of all major muscle groups which are: arms, legs, abdomen, and upper body. It could also involve swimming for 30 minutes, chopping wood, etc.

Aerobic exercise is different from strength training in that it works less with an individuals arm and leg muscles, and works more with the heart and lungs. Both moderate and vigorous aerobic exercises are excellent for burning through stress, raising metabolism, and getting rid of toxins in the body.

Holistic Exercise

A **holistic** activity is one that enhances all levels of a living system simultaneously. Holistic activities for human beings will enhance the health of our body, mind, emotions, and even sense of self. One such activity, that is known for accomplishing all of these measures simultaneously, is QiGong. The physical activity Tai Chi is one of the forms of QiGong but there are many more.

QiGong can be a great activity for improving balance, strength, coordination, and mental/emotional health, all at once. It is very relaxing, and has been referred to as "meditation in motion." QiGong can be considered both an exercise and a relaxation technique.

If you would like to explore QiGong, I would highly recommend Robert Peng's QiGong DVDs, which are purchasable on several websites.

Other forms of exercise can also be made more holistic by focusing one's attention on the breath or body while in motion. This practice can lead to an improved mind/body connection.

Movement and Burn-Out

If a person is already feeling burnt-out from chronic stress, then exercise may be one of the last things that they want to engage in. They may feel too tired to begin.

For this person, simply walking can be a great form of stress-release and exercise, if nothing else seems appealing. This person may even find that a little movement can help them to revive some lost energy. I once heard a friend say it this way: "Energy begets energy."

Pillar 4 ~ Social Support

Have you ever had a friend or family member you knew you could turn to in times of either joy or sadness, and things always seemed to get better after meeting up with them? Or maybe for you, after a distressing day at work, there's a lovable pet that you know you can turn to for some cuddles. Emotional and mental support in the form of a nurturing support system is absolutely a cornerstone of stress management. Unless you are a monk or a mountain man living out in the woods alone, and you know for sure that this is your calling, having a strong support system will be paramount for managing stress in the ever-changing digital age that we now find ourselves in.

Social support is not only a pillar that I've identified in managing stress, it's also part of a book titled *The Depression Cure*. The author, Dr. Stephen S. Ilardi has identified social support as being a key factor in recovering from depression.

Social support can alleviate symptoms of both depression and stress in several ways. For one, being around friends and family helps us to get 'out of our heads' and into the present moment. We can leave any stressful rumination that we may be doing behind and possibly talk to people about how we are feeling. Alternatively, we may choose to just lighten up and have a good time.

Second, being around people that we enjoy spending time with causes a feeling of bonding which leads to a release of the hormone **oxytocin**. Oxytocin is known for being released when a mother bonds to her child, when partners bond in relationships, and when friends come together. For this reason, scientists nickname it "the love hormone." When oxytocin is released into the blood stream during times of bonding, it has been found to lower blood pressure and cortisol levels.

The third, but certainly not the final way, that a good support system lowers distress is by giving people an opportunity to relate to others and share in challenges and struggles.

As mentioned earlier, it has been found that societies where people routinely live to the age of 100 all have strong social bonds. These societies tend to place a lot of value on togetherness. It has also been found that in villages around the world where people still practice hunting and small farming, that individuals living in the village generally have much better mental health than people living in the United States. The fact that Americans often look at primitive villages as "backward" or "un-developed" shows that we don't yet understand the value of sound mental health and togetherness.

In the United States and much of the developed world, technology and screens have filled our lives, and made many things easier to accomplish. It's also caused individuals to spend more time alone, leading to more distress overall.

Many of the forms of communication that are now preferred happen through the use of technology such as texting, email, and other forms of instant messaging. These forms of communication, which so often come into play because we miss being around others, are not good replacements for face-to-face social bonding. They simply don't give people the release of oxytocin and feelings of comfort that can come from good old fashioned social gatherings. On top of that, instant messaging can lead to either improper conveyance, or understanding, of what is being said. If so, stress and frustration will only increase.

If one chooses to use technology as a tool to stay connected with others, either video messaging or talking over the phone is much better for bonding than instant text messaging. Video and voice calls can allow two people to feel some level of connection, even across the globe.

Finding Your Tribe

If you are a person who consistently finds yourself being alone, I don't mean to bum you out or make you think that you are doing something wrong. I just want to highlight the point that a good social support network will be a great help in managing stress. If you already know of people that you could spend more time with and who will support you, I would encourage you to reach out to them. If not, then it's time to find your tribe.

Your 'tribe' is a group of people with interests similar to yours, whom you enjoy being around, simply because it feels good to do so.

Following some of the advice in Pillar 2 on *Doing What You Love* can actually be a good starting point in finding your tribe. If you can identify what your top interests are and pursue activities that you love doing, you will likely meet others to share in that enjoyment with. This will be especially true if those activities force you to get out from behind a screen and into social settings.

Relationship Building

Relationship building is all about forming new, healthy friendships, and making the most out of the relationships that one already has in place. The process of relationship building is generally enjoyable, although initially, it can feel uncomfortable if a person isn't used to expressing their personality.

Say, for example, you are aware of a gathering of people with like interests as yours that you could attend. It can feel uncomfortable and awkward at first to join that group, especially if you are alone and everyone at the gathering already knows one another. It can feel a bit like being the new kid in class. It can also be challenging to initiate conversations with people you haven't met, especially if you find yourself being more introverted. If you can feel the discomfort that meeting new people can bring, and then push forward and do it anyway, you will likely make some new friends and social contacts.

The process of relationship building is also very rewarding to practice with the relationships that one already has in place. Friendships can be enhanced considerably by letting the people in your life know that you appreciate them, for example.

What follows are some of the key elements of relationship building. They can be applied to both making new contacts and strengthening current bonds.

- <u>Be Yourself</u>. In order to make good quality social connections you will have to be your true and authentic self. Everyone is unique and there are several people in this world who will appreciate your uniqueness. If you don't express yourself authentically, on the other hand, then no one can be friends with the *real you*.
- <u>Listen Deeply</u>. When a friend is speaking, rather than being on your phone or in your mind, listen to what they are saying.
- <u>Express Yourself</u>. Nobody wants to talk to a wall… It's boring. If you are true to yourself and then express your uniqueness, you will be far more interesting. Make no mistake about it, some people will not really like the true

expression of *you*, but the ones who do will like you a lot. I have many friends who express themselves truly and are weird, but they are "my type of weird."

- <u>Accept Different Views</u>. This is a big one. I know many people who build a lot of walls between themselves and others, because they are only willing to make friends with people who have the exact same views and opinions as they do.

  Some views people have will be too off-putting to overcome. A person who is a neo-nazi, let's say, is not one that I can be friends with. On the other hand, if you consider yourself a democrat or republican, be willing to make friends with people who have a different allegiance than yours. Build as few walls as possible.

- <u>Express Appreciation</u>. If you already have good social contacts in your life, appreciate these people, and let them know it. My wife is great at this. She frequently lets her friends and family know that she is thankful for their connection. I like to follow her lead and thank her for both loving me and putting up with me.

- <u>Treat Yourself Well</u>. The dynamics of our relationships often reflect how we treat our *own* selves. If you treat yourself well, others are likely to do the same.

- <u>Forgive</u>. All of the best relationships that I've had in my life included the element of forgiveness. I am not perfect, nor was the other person, but we were willing to forgive each other for our shortcomings. If we were annoyed with one another, we may need some time apart, but then coming back together we could talk things through. Forgiveness is very rewarding, and necessary to make strong bonds.

Gender Differences During Distress

Men and women exhibit slightly different behaviors in response to mental/emotional distress. Both genders go into the 'fight or flight mode,' but women have also demonstrated a tendency to nurture, support, and bond during times of distress. This tendency that women demonstrate to nurture, support, and bond- especially with one another- has been nicknamed 'tend and befriend' behavior.

The reason that men and women exhibit slightly different behaviors in response to distress is likely due to human history and adaptation. In hunter-gatherer times, it was more likely for men to be in dangerous circumstances. This could be during a hunt, a feud, or a battle with a neighboring tribe. As such, when men are triggered into the 'fight or flight' mode it's more common for them to demonstrate either angry or aggressive behavior.

Women during hunter-gatherer times were more likely to band together in the village and take care of the young during times of distress. So when the stress response is triggered in modern times, women can certainly still get hostile but are more likely than men to talk things out and to reach for social support.

On top of that, men in Western Culture are raised and encouraged to hide their emotions and always act 'tough' - even when they are angry, sad, or bitter. It's truly a great disservice we are doing to boys and men, in this day and age, in not letting them express how they are really feeling.

For reasons both cultural and adaptive, a woman is more likely to express her emotions and to seek help in times of chronic stress. In today's world, this behavior is by far healthier. 'Tend and befriend' behavior is an excellent coping strategy in dealing with either short-term, or chronic, distress.

As a man, I still find it hard at times to ask for help, and to seek support when I'm going through distress… Even though I understand the importance and value of doing so. That being said, ever since my sister passed away, and I found myself faced with both grief and trauma, I've made a real commitment to adapting healthier support behaviors.

These days, if I'm going through something really hard, and I can't overcome it on my own, I will reach out for mental health support. I am also more likely, now, to tell people how I am feeling.

I find these self-care measures very valuable for two reasons: One, it feels good to 'vent' my feelings, and I am often met with compassion after doing so. Two, I set a better example for the men and boys around me. It's possible, as a man, to evolve how we respond to mental/emotional distress.

Asking For Help

Asking for help can be a difficult thing. Many of us go through life with an "I can do everything on my own" mentality. But of course, we people can't do everything on our own. We need people. And we need help.

So we will need to learn to ask for help in several areas of our lives: with physical chores, with work, with family or household duties, and with our mental and emotional health.

In the case of mental and emotional health, there are several resources a person can turn to for assistance. If our issue isn't debilitating or very serious, then we can simply turn to a trusted friend or mentor to talk out our struggles with. If the mental and emotional stress we are facing is overbearing, then we should seek help from a qualified therapist, counselor, or mental health coach. A counselor at your workplace, school, or in a community can be a good person to turn to for **talk therapy**.

In my work as a health coach, I also give people a safe environment to talk about their stressors, but then I help them to adopt new behaviors to better manage stress.

At times, I know that a client's issues with mental and emotional health are outside of my abilities to assist. If, for example, you are feeling severe discomfort from emotional stress, are carrying around heavy trauma, or feel like you can't go on, then you should seek to find a suitable therapist. Plain and simple.

Asking for help can also come in the form of asking your social group to help you with a move, chores, or household duties. Consider who supports you, and who you could ask for help in your personal life. Are you doing too much at work or home while others are doing very little? It may be time to begin explaining to people how you feel and asking for assistance. If so, even if others do not perform a task as well as you, consider the value of letting go and trusting others to help you. This is called either **out-sourcing** or **delegating**.

If you receive help from people outside of your home or work then when they need help, do your best to be there *for them*. If you can already see that they need assistance with something, then offer to help them before they even ask. If you have a good friend that you occasionally turn to in order to talk through your struggles, then be there for them when they need it.

Conflict Resolution

Conflicts with other people are an almost inevitable part of life. In marriage, at work, with family, with friends, and in relationships of all kinds, conflicts will happen. Conflicts also happen between groups of people and obviously between nations.

Living life in a state of conflict *stinks*. Conflict causes distress, and many of people's top stressors come from interpersonal conflicts. Luckily, there are sound ways to resolve conflicts.

There are two fields of study, which I'm aware of, which help people to resolve conflicts between themselves and others (these techniques could even be applied for group conflict). The two fields of study are NVC (Non-Violent Communication) and Assertiveness Training. These skills do not usually come naturally to people and it's hard to find people who deal with conflict well, so learning these skills can be really beneficial.

Whenever we feel conflict in an interpersonal relationship, it will trigger mental/emotional distress. If the conflict is physically abusive, then obviously that will add an element of physical distress. But most conflicts aren't physical in nature. Most relationship conflict is caused by an individual feeling either insulted, used, under-appreciated, or feeling that their needs are unmet in a relationship. According to Assertiveness Training, there are three different "styles" which people adopt for dealing with conflicts. They are:

1. **Passive**. This style of behavior comes from an individual feeling too frightened or uncomfortable to address a conflict. This style leads to an individual 'holding things in' and not saying anything so that they can avoid confrontation. In cases where the person(s) we are in conflict with could hurt or kill us, this style may *need* to be employed. Otherwise, this behavior style is unhealthy, and can lead to feelings of resentment, disgust, or anger within the person who is 'holding things in.' Just like Jim Carrey's character in the movie *Me, Myself, and Irene*, this individual may eventually 'blow up' and express themselves violently. Practicing assertiveness can relieve some of the pressure that this individual is experiencing, so that they won't need to 'blow up' emotionally. The type B and type D personalities described previously are the most likely to employ the passive style in conflict.

2. **Aggressive**. This type of behavior is almost opposite to that of the passive style. It involves using intimidation, deceit, or forcefulness to either end or intensify a conflict. In a relationship, the aggressive behavior style could lead to yelling, accusing, or threatening from the aggressor. The aggressive behavior style is more proactive than the

passive style but leads to resentment and loss of trust from the other party. Unbalanced Type A individuals can demonstrate this behavior style.

3. **Assertive**. Assertive behavior is the most constructive and usually the most promising way to deal with conflict. It involves the assertive individual expressing what they feel, why they feel that way, and what they hope can be done to resolve the conflict. Assertive behavior may make the other person(s) uncomfortable, but that is not the goal. The goal is to find a constructive resolution to a conflict. Often, when one person is assertive but not aggressive, the other person will feel able to voice their own frustrations so that understanding and compromise can be achieved.

Questions to Consider

1. Which behavior style do you most often demonstrate in conflicts: passive, aggressive, or assertive? And why?
2. Are there people who make you feel upset, whom you could talk to about these feelings to relieve some distress
3. Are there conflicts in your life that could be resolved with a constructive conversation and expression of feelings?

Practicing Assertiveness

For stress management, learning to be assertive is a great skill to have. Being too passive can leave an individual with unresolved resentments leading to a lot of pent-up and unresolved emotional distress. Being too aggressive can create distrust and anger from other people, and also make us feel on edge.

The intention of being assertive is to resolve conflicts in the most peaceful way possible. Being assertive helps us to establish healthy boundaries and to declare how we expect to be treated.

If you have a conflict going on between you and another person, or you feel upset with someone, then it will be healthy to confront them with how you are feeling. If you can meet with them in person, this will be preferred. When you do, realize that you may feel *very* uncomfortable or upset. Do your best to stay calm and not get aggressive or defensive. Look at them with good eye contact, have a strong posture, and state confidently what behaviors this person has been demonstrating that are causing you to feel upset.

You may want to rehearse what you will say ahead of time, but don't spend too long rehearsing because you may get into an entire argument in your mind that never actually ends up happening.

Confront this person or people as soon as possible. If you feel too upset or scared to meet this individual in person, then you may wish to send a message to this person through technology, but remember to follow the principles of constructive assertiveness.

After letting the person know what behavior is upsetting you, also let them know how you are feeling. Do your best here to use "I" statements. For example, you may say, "You haven't done this yet, and *I* feel this way about it." If you say, "you make me feel this way," or "you always do this," the person may feel attacked and go on the defensive.

After stating the behavior you feel uncomfortable with and how it makes *you* feel with an "I" statement, make a request. This could sound something like, "could you please do it this way next time," or, "I would really like you to show up tomorrow," "or "I NEED you to respect me more in this area." The word "need" will give the strongest request.

If the person wants to make a reply to your statement, then listen intently. If they feel upset, or go on the defensive, you could say something like, "Hey, relax, I'm just trying to reach a resolution on this." Be willing to reach a compromise, in most cases, but don't sacrifice anything that you feel you need to happen.

When I've practiced assertiveness in my life, I've found it to work wonders. If I can explain how I am feeling effectively, then the person that I'm in conflict with will often be understanding and considerate. I've used assertiveness on managers and authority figures and found them to be more reasonable people than I expected.

I'm sure that there are a few unreasonable people in the world, but practicing assertiveness has always gone well in my experience. Give it a try. Don't underestimate the power of constructive assertiveness. It can work wonders and resolve long-held distress.

The Content of an Assertive Message

1. Point out the behavior	2. Explain how the behavior affects you	3. State what you need to happen
When you don't respond,...	...I feel like I'm being ignored.	I need to know you're listening.
When you're late to the office,...	...I have to handle your calls.	I need you to be on time for now on.
When you ask me the same question over and over,...	...I feel you don't believe I've made a final decision.	I need you to realize I'm not going to change my mind.

Yes or No?

In life, we will receive many opportunities that we can either say "yes" or "no" to. Many of these opportunities will come to us through a request made by others.

Saying yes to opportunities, and life, can be a very rewarding decision to make. Saying yes to opportunities gives us the possibility to grow, learn, and to enjoy the opportunities which we say yes to. On the other hand, if you find yourself saying yes to too many requests, it can leave you feeling drained and stretched thin.

If you are receiving a lot of requests from people, remember that for balanced-healthy-living you will likely need to say no in certain circumstances. This will create boundaries in your life and make you feel more confident and assertive.

If you find that you've already said yes to too many things and are already worn thin, then it may be time to re-assess. Are there things in your life that you would like to do less of, so that you can free up time for other priorities? If so, then consider how you could have conversations with people to let them know that you would like to scale back on these duties. Be assertive.

Nurturing Relationships

Good quality relationships- that are nurturing- will certainly be more life-enhancing than poor ones. A relationship that creates more distress than it relieves will eventually crumble. One, or both, parties will want to leave it behind.

A nurturing relationship will be one that you can turn to either in times of need for support or in times of joy for celebration. Nurturing relationships will include trust, openness, honesty, and respect. In a nurturing relationship, you will feel comfortable being yourself as much as possible. The other person will either appreciate your openness, or at least respect you. You don't have to agree on everything.

In a nurturing relationship, both people will respect each other's desires and goals. There will likely be mutual support and encouragement

Poor relationships, on the other hand, are missing one or more of these qualities. These unhealthy relationships are perhaps better than having no friends at all, but should not be favored.

If you have people in your life that you know you have good relationships with, then enjoy those relationships as much as possible. The qualities of nurturing relationships, which include: trust, openness, honesty, respect, and support are gifts that you can give to others. If you do present these gifts in a relationship, it will be similar to watering and nurturing a plant (a 'relationship tree'), and this plant will grow strong and vital.

Alone Time

For optimal mental and emotional well-being, it's important to balance time around others with a little alone time. The reason that relationship building and social support are discussed more in this pillar than the value of alone time, is that forming healthy relationships and getting together with people tends to be more difficult for people than finding alone time.

Alone time is different than *loneliness*. Loneliness is an emotion that people associate with being alone. Loneliness can actually be felt when we are surrounded by others if we feel like we don't 'jive' with the group.

Cultivating the ability to be alone with ourselves without feeling lonely, can be very valuable for uncovering our true desires, calming our minds, and relaxing. Most of the methods for *Triggering Relaxation* in Pillar 1 involve being alone. Spending time alone allows us to reset ourselves and to truly enjoy our friends and family when we see them again.

The most productive ways to spend alone time may include journaling, reading, learning, triggering relaxation, or reflecting on our experiences. A person who is capable of both being alone and spending their alone time productively, will be a well-balanced force in this world.

Pillar 5 ~ The Art of Eating

Eating a good meal that is full of yummy foods can be calming to the nervous system and relaxing to the mind and body. Eating a wholesome meal with friends and family is a great way to both enjoy one another's company and to celebrate the food being consumed.

In general, there are four elements to the eating experience:

1. Where to Eat
2. When to Eat
3. What to Eat
4. How to Eat

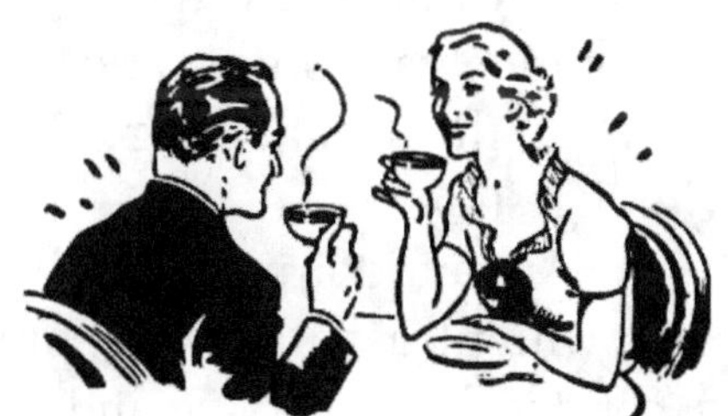

Eating for stress management is all about getting each element of the eating experience as close to optimal as possible. Missing the mark on any one of these elements can cause undue stress to the body (physical distress) and lead to indigestion and chronic inflammation.

The Art of Eating is all about treating the eating experience itself as an art form, which means that the more you practice optimal eating, the better you will get at it. The Art of Eating involves savoring and reveling in the eating experience, and turning it into a practice that rejuvenates the mind, body, and spirit.

We will discuss each element of the eating experience in order and how to get each element as close to optimal as possible. Since there seem to be a million books on diet and nutrition currently on the market, we will not touch on *what to eat* extensively. We will pay special attention to the fourth element of eating- how you eat- since people under chronic stress often eat hurriedly and digest their food poorly.

Where to Eat

Choosing an environment for eating that is as soothing and as calming as possible will be best for practicing the art of eating. On the other hand, eating in an environment that is loud, chaotic, or frantic can actually put the body and mind into a state of distress and is not conducive to digesting and assimilating food. One of my mentors, Dr. Liis Mattik used to say it this way: "Nobody can digest food at a rock concert."

The place where you eat should be chosen based on how well it will help you to digest your meal. If the environment is soothing and calming, then the body is likely to go into the 'rest and digest' mode, which obviously helps with digestion.

An outdoor patio can be a great place to eat. A dining room with pleasant lighting, pretty flowers, and soft music will be conducive to relaxing and digesting.

If a person does have to eat at work (we've all been there), then actions to make the environment as calming as possible can be taken. This will mean pausing all work activities, possibly putting in some headphones with piano music, and going somewhere as quiet as possible.

Another aspect of where one eats involves who is there… It's preferable to eat with people that you know, like, and trust. People that are boisterous, complaining, or judging the meal negatively will not help with optimal eating.

The two best options are to either eat with people that you like, or to eat alone. People that you enjoy being around can make a meal both jovial and relaxing.

When to Eat

If a person is under a lot of distress, then eating a nutritious breakfast before 10:00 a.m. will be crucial, because this individual is constantly burning through their energy reserves and will almost certainly feel sluggish without breakfast. For everyone else, eating a nutritious breakfast will still be beneficial. Eating breakfast has been linked to the balancing of blood sugar, greater energy and focus, and even improved weight management. Good breakfast foods include oatmeal, nuts, raisins, toast, fruit, or eggs. Breakfast should be eaten, but not so much, that you ruin your appetite for lunch.

A good hearty lunch (eaten between 11:00 a.m. and 1:00 p.m.) should ideally be your biggest meal of the day. This is because the human body's ability to digest and assimilate food is highest at midday. For managing stress, lunch should never be skipped unless one is sick or fasting. A good noon-time meal will consist of a combination of proteins, fats, and carbohydrates.

Around 3:00 to 4:00 p.m. cortisol levels will naturally dip, leaving many individuals feeling sleepy. If a snack like trail mix, a small smoothie, or some snack bars can be eaten at this time, it may help to revive you until the evening.

Dinner (aka supper, depending on where you live) is a great time to gather everyone together for a nice meal. Finishing dinner as early in the evening as possible (ex: 6:00 p.m.) will be optimal for overall health. This will give the body appropriate time to digest and relax before bed time.

What to Eat

What to eat should be decided with taste in mind. Tasteful food is comforting and is enjoyable to the senses. That being said, *some* tasteful food is hard for the body to process and adds physical distress, whereas other tasteful food is life-enhancing and healing for the body.

There are a lot of theories on diet in this day and age. There are constantly changes being made as to what constitutes a healthy diet versus an unhealthy diet.

Specifically, the best diet for managing stress is the one that places the least distress on your body and mind. And how do you know what diet is least distressing and best for you? That can be discovered by treating eating as an experiment and paying close attention to how you <u>feel</u> after eating.

You can have the mindset that your body is a laboratory. Every time you eat or drink something, it's like conducting an experiment. Pay close attention to how you are feeling after consuming each food or drink. This will tell you the results of your eating experiments. Notice after eating if you are belching, feeling heavy, having acid indigestion, or any other symptoms. You can even record what you eat and drink and how you feel afterward if you like. This is called **food journaling**.

If you do have any of the symptoms named previously (belching, feeling heavy, etc.) you likely ate too much or ate food that was not optimal for your body at this time.

If you want to limit physical distress, then eat foods that leave your body feeling good after eating them. If you have a food allergy or sensitivity to anything like milk, wheat, dairy, nuts, peppers, etc. then do your best to avoid these foods. Food sensitivities create inflammation in the body, and take a lot of energy to rebalance.

Also, for minimizing distress, favor foods that are as natural and as minimally processed as possible. Good ol' fruits, vegetables, beans, nuts, and fresh meats will have more nutrients and fewer chemical additives than processed foods.

Caffeine and processed sugar are two substances that people love to reach for if they are feeling fatigued from distress. The trouble with these substances, is that they can fuel the 'fight or flight' response and leave people trapped in a vicious cycle. Natural sugars from fruits will be better than processed sugars, and if caffeine is consumed, green or black tea will usually be healthier than coffee.

One of the interesting things about a good diet, is that it will affect not only how your body looks and feels, but also how you feel emotionally. There is a strong link between food and mood. Vitamins and nutrients (such as vitamin C, the B vitamins, and selenium) are needed for the production of **'happy hormones'** in the body such as serotonin and dopamine. Good food promotes a good mood.

How to Eat

Eating in a calm and relaxed manner while being aware of the sensory pleasures of food is the best way to eat for optimal digestion and intake of nutrients. It's also the best way to eat for the enjoyment of flavor, texture, and taste. Focusing on what is being eaten honors the sacrifice that another living being made so that you may survive, and also gives the greatest opportunity for the intake of nutrition.

If a person is in the 'fight or flight' mode while eating, they will not be able to process their food optimally. The energy and focus of the body simply isn't in the digestive system during these moments. If our ancestors were running from a bear, it's not likely that their body would have wanted to stop and eat.

Here are some suggestions for stress-free eating and proper intake of nutrients:
- Prepare your body for eating by relaxing a bit before a meal.

- Make food choices based on taste, nutrition, and what you've experienced is best for you.
- Definitely sit down while eating.
- When your food arrives, say 'grace' or a thank you before eating. Get in touch with your body. These things can both happen through a prayer.
- Chew your food slowly and thoroughly, noticing the flavors and textures.
- Do your best to eliminate any distractions such as electronics or intense conversations.
- Try not to rush. Even if you only have 15 minutes to eat, eliminating any distractions and eating alone can maximize the time which you do have.
- Sit for at least 5 minutes after your meal is finished.
- If you have time to walk, a short walk after a meal can be a great way to relax and to aid digestion.

Pillar 6 ~ Managing Time & Money

Psychologists assess people's stress levels by conducting Perceived Stress Surveys. Two of the top stressors that are consistently reported by people taking perceived stress surveys are: feeling pinched for time, and financial concerns. As such, learning how to manage both time and money will be a crucial element of every person's stress management journey. Time, money, and feelings of either relaxation or distress, are all intimately linked.

Time is a pretty fixed element for each person- we each have 24 hours in a day. Money, on the other hand, isn't set. We all have varying amounts of money, with our overall amount tending to fluctuate with time sort of like the seasons. Sometimes we may feel like we are doing well with time and money management. At other times, we may feel like we are struggling with either one or both.

It's most people's opinion that if they just had more time and money, then everything would be better. Unfortunately, this isn't necessarily the case.

If each person was given an extra four hours in the day, the people who say "yes" to too many options, would most likely end up scheduling-in their extra four hours and would then again feel pinched for time.

If each person was given, let's say, a free $1,000 a month, some people would spend it wisely (or save it), while others would squander it away. On top of that, having a lot of money doesn't mean that a person won't feel stressed about their financial future. Perceived stress levels do indeed go down with more earnings (up to $75,000 annually, per household), but financial fears can still creep into a person's mind, no matter what their earning power. Some people will feel the need to constantly hoard money and resources due to that nagging fear of the unknown and constantly worrying about not having *enough*.

As such, in this part of the reading, we will first discuss how a person can best manage their 24 hours in a day so that they will be set up to feel less distressed and more capable of earning money. We will then talk about money management a bit, and consider how each of us can face our fear over not having *enough*. Even if we as people don't make a lot of money, we can still face our financial worries and manifest peace in this area.

When it comes to time and money, we will all want to learn how to spend both wisely. I like to view the ways that I spend both my time and my money as investments. At times, we will all want to spend time and money on things simply for pleasure and enjoyment. Nothing wrong with that. At other times, we will want to spend our time and money in ways that yield a good return on investment.

Prioritizing

Have you ever heard someone use the expression, "You need to get your priorities straight!" Usually, when people use that expression, what they really want is for another person's priorities to align with how they think that person should live.

Although that expression isn't usually one offered in

either genuine care or kindness, the advice is actually pretty good. To live a fulfilling life, we all need to get our priorities straight.

So far in this book, we have discussed the concepts of both "heartfelt desires" and "doing what one loves." These two concepts will fit in nicely with prioritizing. Prioritizing is all about first considering what we really want to do and experience in life, and then aligning our actions and time expenditure with these desires. Of course, we will also have to balance time spent on things we love doing with our other responsibilities.

The things which we make a top priority for ourselves will likely give us insight into how to best spend our time, and will hopefully lead us to fulfilling our top desires and goals.

Over a lifetime, a person's priorities will change and evolve. A college student's priorities will obviously be very different from an older retired person's. The priorities of someone who lives in Southern California and is into high-fashion will be very different from those of a mountain man hidden in the hills of Montana.

To know how to best spend our time, it's very valuable to consider what our top priorities are. When I've found myself in states of 'chronic rush' with little self-care time, I've had to really sit down and decide how to better spend my time, to make self-care a bigger priority.

Stephen Covey, author of *The 7 Habits of Highly Effective People*, lists "sharpening the saw" as one of the habits of highly successful individuals that he has spoken with. "Sharpening the saw" is all about investing in our overall health with both our time and money, so that we can be effective and "sharp" in the world. In this metaphor, the "saw" represents our mind and body.

<u>**A Prioritizing Exercise**</u>

Take out a piece of paper, and a pen, and write out your top ten priorities. Then label your top three priorities with an A, middle three priorities with a B, and less important things with a C.

You may find that deciding on only three top priorities with an A is challenging. That being said, those three A priorities will end up being what your life pretty much revolves around. If you are a working parent, your career and family will likely each receive A's, and then you will have to decide upon just one more top priority to really place your time and energy upon.

The priorities which get labeled with a B will likely be things that are still pretty important to you, and that you will be able to find time for during the week.

The C priorities are more difficult to find time for. When you sit down to prioritize, you may find that some things which you wish you could find time for don't make it into either the A or B category. These things may then end up receiving little importance or attention in your life.

Sometimes, hard decisions will have to be made, and "friendship time" or "entertainment time," while being very valuable, will have to take a cutback. At other times, we may need to find ways to lessen our work and daily responsibilities, so that we can make time for other priorities that we consider important.

Jen is a Mom of three who finds herself 'spread thin' with all of her responsibilities to her husband, her children, and her part-time job as a nurse. After considering her top priorities, Jen realizes that she is not spending enough time "taking care of self." She also wishes that she and her husband could golf once or twice a week, as they did before having babies. Jen decides that to feed these priorities, her kids will only be able to sign up for one extra-curricular activity at a time and that she will need to hire a sitter for the kids while her and her man go golfing. The multiple activities that two of her kids are in, has caused her to spend too much time driving youngsters around, and not enough time for her own enjoyment.

<u>Jen's Top Priorities:</u>
Family (A), Exercise (B)
Work (A), Children's Activities (B)
Taking Care of Self (A), Wine with Friends (C)
Chores (C), Walking Dog (C)
Journaling (B), Gardening (C)

Screen Time

Rarely when people list their top priorities, do they ever list "Facebook," "Netflix," "Youtube," or "Social Media." Yet, a lot of potential free time is spent (and plenty wasted) engrossed on these sites.

Overall screen time, which includes time spent in front of a computer, cell phone, or iPad has become a big time expenditure in the Digital Age. Learning how to use these sources of technology to enhance our lives, rather than deplete them, will be a key challenge in the 21st century.

If a person can learn to use technology to improve their time management and to help themselves connect with friends and family, then they will be able to use this tool to lessen distress.

Several of the relaxation methods listed earlier in the book can be accessed through the use of technology. I would say that this is a healthy way to take advantage of technological resources.

I have noticed in my life, that I can either use technology to make myself feel more at peace or more distressed. It's up to me. Every person who can access technology, and use it for the enhancement of life, is much more likely to enjoy living in the 21st century.

Screen time and time for sleep are likely the two most malleable aspects of most people's day. If we are spending about 8 hours a day at work or school, plus spending some time eating and meeting with other people, these areas will be pretty much 'set in stone.' What we do with the rest of our day is often up to us.

If you notice yourself spending more than 2 to 3 hours a day looking at a screen for non-work related duties, it may be time to consider how you could better spend that time. You can even do a 'digital detox' for an evening or a weekend where you avoid screen time altogether and see how you feel and respond.

Many people upon seeing their lives get busier will first sacrifice sleep to make extra time for daily activities. Some people will sacrifice sleep in order to enjoy screen time. Sleep is very restorative for body, mind, and emotions and every individual should aim to get 7 to 9 hours of this restorative stuff every night. Sacrificing sleep for a screen is not a great habit to get into.

Overall, if you notice yourself spending a lot of time on a screen during your free time, it may be valuable to cut back on this and to make more time for one of your higher priorities.

Sleep

To accomplish all of one's top priorities, a good sleeping routine will be crucial. Whether or not a person has a successful day, and how they feel during it, are both very dependent on a good night's rest. Sleeping can be a very frustrating part of life for people who don't get enough of it.

Practicing what's called good **sleep hygiene** can help a person to create better sleeping habits, and improve both one's quality and quantity of sleep. There are many ways to improve one's quality of sleep, including, going to bed and waking at similar times each day, not eating a big meal too late at night, managing stress, being active during the day, and leaving 30 to 60 minutes before bed to 'wind down' without any work or electronics. It will also be beneficial to make one's sleeping room as conducive to sleep as possible by having it very dark, cool, and quiet; having a good bed, pillows, and blankets; and possibly running a white noise machine.

Each one of us will benefit majorly from a good **sleeping routine**, and there are constantly ways to improve our sleep hygiene to accomplish just that. More on this can be found by using technology wisely and reading information published by the Sleep Foundation on the world wide web.

According to the Sleep Foundation, several things can impede a good night of sleep. These include drinking caffeine, physical pain, the light from electronics, and excessive alcohol consumption (a person drinking a lot may 'pass out' but the sleep will be of low quality). To get a good night's rest, one should avoid as many impediments to sleep as possible. Avoiding the use of stimulating substances and screen light, will be two valuable steps for most people. Screen light from electronics can actually trick our brains into thinking that it's still daytime and inhibit the release of sleep-promoting hormones.

Some substances can actually help an individual to get a better night's sleep including low-dose melatonin, 5-HTP, or ashwagandha.

Due to the natural daily cycle of cortisol as well as several other hormones, including melatonin, it is most preferable to be in bed when it's dark out between 10 pm to 6 am. This will yield the most restorative rest.

It's also of value to be awake and active during the daylight hours. Being either a 'night owl' or having to work overnights can be very hard on one's mental/emotional health. You would think that sleeping 7 to 9 hours would have the same effect no matter when it happens, but due to our bodies natural daily cycles this simply isn't the case. It's most restorative to be in bed during the night when cortisol levels are low and melatonin levels are high.

That being said, thank goodness that there are people who work overnights at hospitals and in security roles. They are there to aid us when we have emergencies. For these individuals, it will be very important to sleep soon after work, make their sleeping room as dark as possible, and vehemently stick to their sleeping routine.

Scheduling - Putting it All Together

To accomplish all of our top priorities, we will have to plan our days effectively. For this, literally getting a daily planner, notebook, or marker board and setting a schedule can be helpful.

Effective scheduling will be needed to allow one to have enough time to formulate a stress management routine. If you as an individual are feeling a high degree of distress, it will be helpful to begin establishing a routine for stress management immediately.

And it doesn't need to involve a lot of time. Fifteen minutes of meditation or visualization in the morning, plus three 30 minute sessions of movement in the evening, each week, can go a long way. Over time, if you learn how to relax and make your body and mind calm while practicing a relaxation technique, you will eventually be able to go into this state almost at will… even while working or being in a group. This is the pinnacle of stress management, but it will take some time to master.

A lot of time for stress management can be freed up just by giving up a little screen time each day. It is also possible to get creative and do some relaxing while on a break at work or even on a commute in a cab. Relaxing music can be incorporated into more of a person's day for a calming long-term effect.

Whatever your chosen routine of work, enjoyment, and self-care activities, my suggestion would be to be *all there* while doing anything. If you are relaxing, go at it with no distractions. If you are working, get engrossed in what you are doing. If you are with friends and family listen deeply, and share stories. If you are *all there* for each of your activities, you will get as much out of them as possible.

I would also encourage individuals with a Type A personality to not plan-out all of their time during a week. Save some time for spontaneity. Free time on the weekends can be a great time for relaxing, doing something creative, or engaging in a hobby. Spontaneity is all about following our impulses that feel exciting and adventurous.

Managing Money

Money has become such a pervasive item in today's world that many people feel like their lives are run by it. Most people love having money and hate not having it.

Many of us get a message at some point in our lives that money is either "bad" or "evil." We may then have an avoidance to earning money, when in fact, money is neither inherently "good" nor "evil." It's simply a very neutral form of monetary exchange for goods and services. What we do with the money that we make is what counts… For example, we can use it to fuel an addiction that we have, or we can build an orphanage with it to help children.

Money and mental/emotional distress have a bi-directional relationship- not having what a person feels like is *enough* money can lead to distress, and having an excess of mental/emotional distress can make it hard to earn money. Some people even feel distressed about what to do with their money when they have too much of it.

In terms of the relationship between money management and distress, there are basically three components:

1. The actual amount of money that a person has or makes.
2. What a person does with their money.
3. How a person feels about the amount of money they have or make.

The first two components of money management are pretty straight forward. The actual amount of money that a person earns usually comes through either work or good fortune (such as receiving an inheritance).

What a person does with their money is a skill that can be improved to enhance financial stability. This skill has just as big of an impact on financial health as how much money one earns. The third component of money management is the least straight-forward and perhaps the most interesting.

There are a lot of people who make *enough* money, even an abundance of it, but never feel like they have *enough*. They constantly live in a state of worry and distress about not having quite enough money. So in this section, along with discussing how to enhance earnings and how to use them wisely, we will also discuss how to bring this fear out into the light and possibly relieve it.

Earning Money

In this section, I will list some ways that a person can enhance their ability to make money based on my own careful research and experience. Many wealthy individuals have shared what helped them to make their fortunes. Many of these habits are similar from individual to individual.

The habits that wealthy individuals practice, which helped them to earn more money, can be applied and emulated by each of us. Hopefully, we will then have the same success.

1. **Take Care of Your Health**. Being mentally, physically, and emotionally healthy makes it easier to use one's intelligence, be creative, and to be attentive during working hours. This can create the potential to enhance one's earnings.

2. Work on Your **Money Mindset**. What messages did you receive as a child regarding money? Was money hard to come by? Was money evil? Or was money enjoyed, easy

to acquire, and understood as an object which gives oneself the time and freedom to explore what delivers true happiness? The messages which we receive as children regarding money get imprinted on our minds and often affect our earning power as adults. If our parents taught us, and demonstrated, that there is plenty of money in the world, and that we could acquire it easily through persistence, then we are more likely to notice opportunities for the earning of money. The reverse is also true. If you notice yourself constantly feeling like money is "evil" or is "hard to come by" consider investigating new ways of looking at money.

3. **Deepen Some Valuable Skills**. I have had many jobs in my life where I didn't make a lot of money because there were so many other people that could be found to do my job. It made me more replaceable. The people who earn a nice paycheck at their work usually have a set of valuable skills or experience, which makes them more valuable workers. Learning a set of skills that is financially valuable in the world, and then constantly improving these skills, can make a person a very proficient earner of money. This concept can also be synergized with "doing what you love." If you can find some work that you love to do, it will be much easier to consistently practice that work and to get better at it.

4. **Be Open to Receiving Money**. This attitude can help a person to identify more money-making opportunities when they come along. It can also reduce resistance from the sub-conscious mind to allowing money to come to a person for their good efforts.

Using Money Wisely

As mentioned previously, what a person does with their money is just as important as how much money a person earns or has. You can make millions of dollars a year, but even this can disappear quickly if you don't know how to save, spend, and invest it.

A poignant example of this is seen in the world of professional athletics. The jaw-dropping documentary *Broke*, which was released by ESPN, shows how more than half of professional athletes go completely broke after retiring from sports, even though they made millions of dollars during their professional careers. Many of these athletes simply didn't take the time to consider how much money they were making and how much they could spend.

If you don't want to end up like one of these pro athletes, such as Mike Tyson, who made and lost $300 million; then you will need to practice creating a **budget** and **'living within your means**.' Here are several good financial tips that can reduce debt, help with money management, and eventually relieve distress about money:

1. **Budgeting**. Budgeting involves calculating how much money a person earns each month and then figuring out how much can be spent. A good budget will include money for rent, food, clothing, car expenses, insurance, and some fun. After a person decides on a budget, they will know how much they can spend and save each month. Financial advisors state that a good budget will allow a person to save 10% of their earnings each month and put this money into either an emergency fund or a retirement plan. When budgeting and saving, look for areas where you can cut expenses and save money. Some examples may be saving money by eating home-cooked food, canceling under-used subscriptions, and avoiding credit card usage.

2. **Living Within One's Means**. Living within one's means is something that my grandparents taught me when I was young. It's all about making purchasing decisions based on what a person knows that they can afford. Living within one's means makes it possible to

avoid the stress of over-bearing debts by making wise financial choices.

3. **Enjoying Simplicity**. Almost everyone wants to live in a really nice place and own really nice things- nothing wrong with that. That said, there is also a joy and a peace that can be found in living simply. Living simply, or minimally, makes it so that you will have fewer responsibilities, fewer chores, fewer things to care for, and fewer expenses. Living simply may mean that you buy or rent a dwelling that is much cheaper than you can afford, so that you can save money and enjoy little financial strain. The concept of **minimalism** is one that is even becoming popular in the United States, which is basically an extreme commitment to living simply.

4. **Make Good Investments**. If you do make a big investment, or go into debt by making big purchases, that's not necessarily a bad thing. Sometimes you will have to spend money to make money. The key here, is to assess the potential return on investment of your purchase and then to decide if it's worth it. A college education and property are two investments that can yield a good return, if properly chosen. Investing in one's health can also be a good investment. This may involve seeing a chiropractor, taking yoga classes, or receiving counseling. Investments in health can yield peace of mind, pain relief, and years of life.

5. **Educate Yourself**. There are many excellent books for rent at a local library that teach one about money making, investing, and saving. Some of the most popular are: *Think and Grow Rich* by Napolean Hill, Dave Ramsey's *Complete Guide to Money*, and *Rich Dad, Poor Dad* by Robert Kiyosaki. It astounds me how little education is offered to high school students on money management even though this is such a considerable part of life.

6. **Build an Emergency Fund**. Financial advisor and best-selling author Dave Ramsey suggests each family build an emergency fund of $1000 to start out with. This money can yield peace of mind because you know that if you do have an emergency, there will be some money saved to hopefully cover the expenses.

Fear of Not Enough

I used to have a pretty serious fear of heights. Any time that I was either in a mall or on top of a tall building and I looked down at the ground floor below, I would immediately feel myself getting queasy. I would envision how bad it would be if I accidentally fell and plummeted. Of course, this fear was irrational, because I had an immovable railing between myself and the ground below.

Often, people's fears about running out of money and not having enough are just that- fears. Many times, these fears are just as irrational as my fear of heights.

Everyone wants to have enough money to afford their basic needs, plus pay to eat out, do some fun things, and to retire comfortably…

And what is enough? Most financial advisors agree that if an individual or family can pay for all of their basic needs, afford some 'splurges', and still save 10 to 15 percent of their money each month, this is *enough*.

Some people are able to meet all of these measures, but never *feel* like they have enough. They have constant fears surrounding money and no amount of earnings, no matter how vast, can soothe this fear. Watching the news for this person will be a stress trigger, as they hear all of the stories about possible financial collapse, or disarray, that are broadcast each week.

I have also known people that have made very little money, and were consistently just barely skating by, but were never concerned about it. They may even be overspending on unnecessary items each month, but it didn't phase them. For these people, the fear of not enough simply wasn't there.

Me personally, I think that it's wise to save a little money, but I would also like to overcome my fear of never having enough.

The fear of not enough triggers the stress response and the 'fight or flight' mode every time it is felt. Since money constantly needs to be spent on living expenses, a person with a strong fear of not enough can live in an almost perpetual state of distress or anxiety.

If you find yourself with a perpetual fear of not enough, or if you notice yourself having this fear at all, a good thing to do can be to bring these fears to light. Fears are like darkness and they live on being left alone. Bringing them to light involves bringing them out in the open where they can be seen and assessed.

There are many ways of bringing the fear of not enough to light. You could journal about it- write: do I have a fear of not enough and why? Then answer this question for yourself. You can talk about it- by brining up this fear with a good friend, partner, or counselor. Or you can notice when you feel it, and remind yourself that you will be just fine. You have faced financial concerns before, and you ended up being just fine. You will be fine again.

Part 4

How to Manage Stress

26

"Expect great things to come!"
-Anonymous

Putting It All Together

Managing stress is an art form that any person can improve at with practice. Just like any art form, there are individuals who have even mastered this discipline. The people who master stress management have several qualities that they develop over time, which tend to be the same from one master to the next.

People who improve at, and then master stress management, tend to be very aware of their body, mind, and emotions. Rather than letting their thoughts and emotions run on auto-pilot, they become aware of exactly what they are thinking and how this is affecting them. They may then find ways to produce more optimistic or calming thoughts when need be. Masters of managing stress learn how to distract themselves in healthy ways when their thoughts are anxious or stressful.

People who master stress management know how to have fun. They know that fun isn't just something that kids do, or which adults wait for the weekend to experience. They understand that fun and enjoyment are health- and life-enhancing feelings and know how to make fun a part of every day.

People who master stress management go through the ups and downs of life, and they learn how to navigate the down periods with grace. They know how to ask for help when life becomes too heavy.

People who master stress management have a calm and peaceful presence. Other people who wish to live in peace and balance will naturally seek their company.

Mastering the discipline of stress management isn't the norm in today's world, but it is always possible. I have had the fortune of knowing a handful of people like this. These people have reminded me that even if life gets cloudy or stormy, the sun *will* shine again.

At this point, we will now reflect on the journey we have gone on in this book and look to integrate stress management practices into daily life. If you want to improve your skill in this area, reflect on each question or use the questions as journaling topics.

What have you learned about stress management from your own life experience?
(Introduction, A Personal Journey)

What activities or circumstances help you to have fun, feel engaged, or put you in the flow state?
(Part 1, Chapter 2)

Are you aware of when you feel distressed and what triggers it?
(Part 1)

What could you do to live with more balance?
(Part 2, Chapter 12)

Can you learn to pursue your desires while also enjoying life in the present? (Part 2, Chapter 15 & 16)

What positive aspects of your personality can you call upon to feel less distressed, happier, and more at peace?
(Part 2, Chapter 16)

How can you influence the culture(s) of which you are a part in a positive way?
(Part 2, Chapter 17)

What would you like to do more of in life?
(Part 3, Chapter 21)

What types of physical activity do you love doing just for fun?
(Part 3, Chapter 22)

Who in your life helps you to feel more relaxed? Who can you go to for support?
(Part 3, Chapter 23)

How can you make your eating experience more conducive to relaxation?
(Part 3, Chapter 24)

How can you improve your sleep hygiene?
(Part 3, Chapter 25)

What fears do you have, and how could you bring them 'into the light' for soothing?

Would you like to coach yourself?
(Next Section)

Self Coaching

As a Certified Health Coach, I give people a safe environment to voice their health challenges, and to then vent their frustrations and concerns in regards to their specific challenge. I then guide people through exercises and ask them powerful questions, so that they can discover how to better approach their challenge(s). Sometimes through this process, people either discover new ways of looking at their challenges or better ways to view what is happening in their lives. I call these **mindset shifts**.

At other times, people feel called to make a behavior change or to practice a new technique, such as those for relaxation described in Pillar 1 of this book. I can also give individuals my own suggestions that they can apply if they like, or if they feel stuck. Obviously, suggestions from others aren't available when we coach ourselves.

The process of behavior change can involve some ups and downs but is generally very rewarding. Unlike a sports coach who often scolds his athletes when they falter, I always encourage people to be compassionate and kind to themselves as they adopt new behaviors.

I have noticed over time, that I can use my coaching method to coach my own self with some benefit and success. Here I will explain how you can do the same, as it relates specifically to stress management.

The coaching method that I follow is called The CORE Coaching Method. CORE stands for Challenge, Outcome, Reframe, and Envision. It involves going through a process of discovery where a person first describes their Challenge. They then talk about the Outcome that they are experiencing due to their challenge. We will then discuss how a person would rather be feeling, and what it would mean for this person to feel better. The Reframe portion of my coaching method is all about discovering what a person could do to either look at their challenge in a healthier way, or what they could do to make a positive change.

It is then discussed how a person can adopt these changes that they want to make to their lives (Envision) and how any potential setbacks can be navigated and overcome.

Here I will list some questions that you can answer for yourself in order to gain some clarity on your challenge(s), and to brainstorm what you can do differently to help yourself feel some relief. These coaching questions are designed specifically for the process of improved stress management and fit in nicely with the knowledge available in this book.

I would strongly suggest that you pull out some paper and a writing tool to answer these questions, as you go through the process of self-coaching. Writing tends to have a way of connecting thoughts, mind, and intuition that thinking alone can not achieve.

You may be surprised at what you discover. During the process of CORE coaching, people often experience insights or breakthroughs in their thinking that they were not expecting to have.

<u>Challenge</u>
- What is your top stressor at the moment?
- Would you rank your mental/emotional distress as low, medium, or high? Why?
- Do you receive any distress from your environment?
- Are you under distress physically?
- What is your goal for how you'd like to feel?

Identify one main stressor and then proceed to the following steps…

<u>Outcome</u>
- How is this stressor affecting you? (In your journal, write as much as you can about this stressor with the intention to really let out your feelings. At times, journaling can be a very effective coping mechanism.)
- How would you feel if this stressor wasn't in your life?
- When was a time in your life that you felt very good, and low on distress? What was going on in your life at the time?

<u>Reframe</u>
- What is one thing you could start doing differently to relieve the stressor that you are facing?
- What could you start doing to better manage distress as it arises in your life?
- What helps you to feel relaxed?
- Is there a way that you could look at your stressor to make it feel less burdensome?

<u>Envision</u>
After identifying one action step or mindset shift you could make, answer the following questions…
- What will adopting this change look like?
- When can you start, and how will you make time for this new action step?
- How will you feel as a result of this new action?
- How will you measure your success?

- What obstacle(s) could you run into in regards to making this new action a reality?
- How will you overcome this obstacle?

- Who will support you in making this change?
- Who could hold you accountable to your new commitment(s)?

27

Looking Forward

The stress response can have somewhat of an addictive quality. This is because it makes us feel energized, alive and focused for a short time. Many Americans have fallen into the lap of this addition as it's been believed that hard work, striving, and stress will eventually lead a person to feeling accepted, successful, and fulfilled.

But this is an empty promise, and the stress response can eventually leave a person feeling empty.

It's been my tried and true experience that true fulfillment is found through balanced living and enjoyment of life in the present. Balancing one's mind, body, and time can lead a person to having good health, mental proficiency, and an abundance of energy. People with these qualities are very capable of also creating financial success for themselves. It's been found that many of the most financially successful people *do indeed* understand the importance of balance and will practice techniques to help themselves achieve inner balance such as meditation, or yoga, or set aside time for prayer and reflection every day.

Some people who practice stress management and balanced living will even want to push towards mastery, as I described it earlier. This can lead to inner peace, mental calm, and excellent physical functioning.

There is likely no limit to the human potential for balance, peace, and calm. This is because there is likely no limit to the capabilities of the human brain when it comes to intelligence, creativity, memory, and learning. As a people, we just have't gotten to witness the fullness of our potential just yet.

Over time, effectively practicing stress management can really change a person. A person who practices stress management can even heal what psychologists refer to as the **inner child**. This aspect of ourselves can then begin to express itself into the world in a healthy way. Then the qualities of curiosity, liveliness, care, and excitement- all qualities of a healthy child- will merge with our adult selves.

It's possible for a person living in a balanced state to gain more purpose in their lives. The fog which stress and anxiety creates in the mind is lifted, and what a person truly loves to do is eventually noticed and felt. Through the practice of doing what one loves, a person feels energized and inspired. This inspiration may lead a person to using their gifts and excitements to help others; thereby adding more purpose and meaning to one's life.

There are several common personality qualities that one will begin to develop through successful stress management and the overcoming of challenging experiences. Some of the most common ones are light-heartedness, resilience, love, and peace.

Light-Heartedness

A light-hearted person has a calm, happy, and non-serious attitude. In many ways, seriousness is the opposite of light-heartedness, and when people live in a state of fear and stress it's easy to become <u>very</u> serious. A light-hearted attitude is one developed through relaxation and joy, and people demonstrating this quality can become very magnetic.

Resilience

When people successfully overcome challenges, resilience is naturally developed. This makes a person more capable of taking on the next challenge. These people can uplift others during challenging times.

Love

It's been said that "love gives us wings." Living in a calm state makes it easier to fall in love with oneself and all of life. This love can then be shared with others by showing kindness and compassion.

Peace

A person who knows how to balance themselves, knows how to achieve homeostasis. In homeostasis, a condition of mental peace and calm is naturally experienced. For this person, no matter how turbulent the waters of life become, they know that they can always return to peace.

These personality qualities, when they start to be developed, can lift a person into kind of an upward spiral… Practicing stress management leads a person to developing more positive personality qualities, and then embodying these qualities makes it easier to manage stress… and it can go on and on like this.

A person who practices effective stress management and becomes more balanced can become an inspiration for others. It's noticed that this person is feeling light and happy and others will not surprisingly want this for themselves. This balance is then a gift that the peaceful person offers to a world that is really in need of it.

It's my hope that many of us begin to 'go against the grain' and reach for inner peace and balance. This peace may eventually become infectious and everyone else will want to join in. Then the world can become a place so lovely to live in that its hard to imagine, and the youth can learn to live their entire lifetimes in a state of balance.

Thank You

Appendix A: The Anatomy and Physiology of Stress Management

The **human nervous system** is in charge of triggering either the stress response during times of threat or the relaxation response during times of safety. It is composed of the brain, spinal cord, and the nerves that extend from the brain and spinal cord.

The nervous system is very much in charge of communication throughout the body. The brain is like the control center, the conscious/thinking mind is the controller, and the nerves are sort of like fiber optic lines which send messages to all of the trillions of workers in the body (cells). The way that the cells function is dependent on how the nervous system directs them to function.

The human nervous system consists of two divisions by definition: the central nervous system composed of the brain, spinal cord, and optic nerves; and the peripheral nervous system which consists of all the nerves that extend from the central nervous system.

The **peripheral nervous system** is then further divided into the voluntary (or somatic) nervous system and the involuntary (or autonomic) nervous system. The **somatic nervous system** is activated when our mind instructs the limbs of the body to move about, and this is why it is termed voluntary. The **autonomic nervous system** is *automatically* run by the sub-conscious brain without our conscious control, although we *can* learn techniques to influence this division of the nervous system.

The autonomic nervous system is the communication network in charge of maintaining homeostasis within the body. It is also in charge of triggering the 'fight or flight' response in times of threat or the 'rest and digest' mode in times of safety and relaxation.

Stress and The Human Nervous System

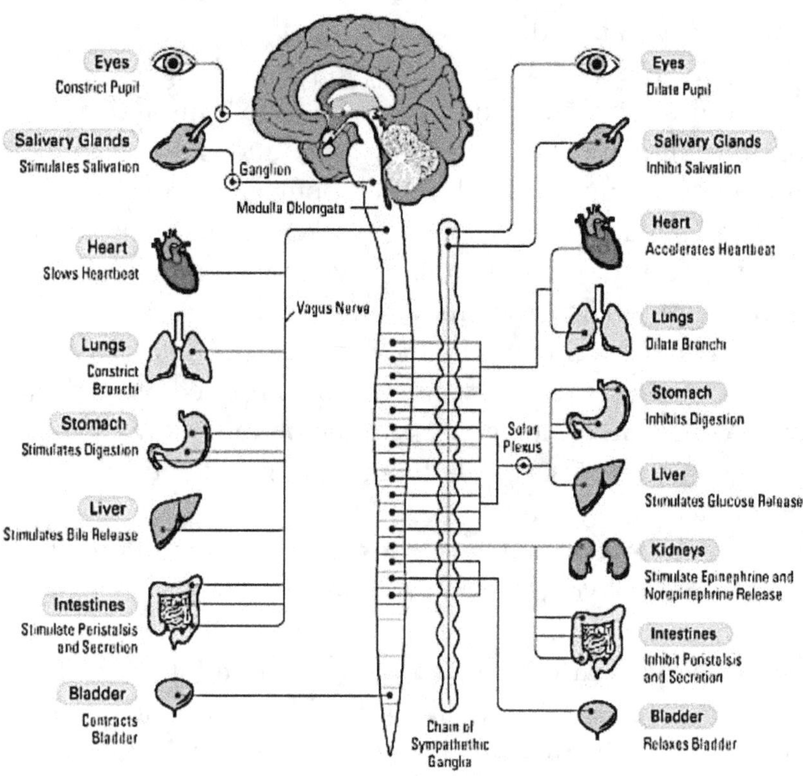

The autonomic system triggers sympathetic nervous system response when threats must be dealt with, and parasympathetic nervous system response when it is perceived acceptable to relax, restore, and heal.

Glossary

Accountability Partners People in your social circle who will help you stay committed and accountable to your goals, habits, and desired behaviors.

Addiction The compulsive engagement in a rewarding behavior even though that behavior has adverse consequences.

Adrenaline A hormone secreted by the adrenal glands, especially in conditions of stress, which increases rates of blood circulation, breathing, and carbohydrate metabolism and prepares muscles for exertion.

Adrenal Fatigue A condition where a person feels very tired and fatigued due to the adrenal glands under-producing a variety of hormones, including cortisol. This condition is normally preceded by chronic stress.

Anxiety A nervous disorder accompanied by excessive worry or panic.

Blue Zones Areas of the world where people live the longest and healthiest lives. These findings come from National Geographic writer Dan Buettner. The five specific blue zones that Buettner discovered are Okinawa, Japan; Sardinia, Italy; Nicoya, Costa Rica; Ikaria, Greece, and Loma Linda, California.

Budget An estimate of income and expenditure over a given period of time.

Burn-Out A state of mental and/or physical exhaustion brought about by chronic stress.

Catastrophizing Using the conscious mind to perform incessant worry.

Chemical Re-Balancing The process of getting accustomed to living in a more relaxed state which leads to changes in hormonal balance. Can be accompanied with some uncomfortable side effects.

Chronic Stress Negative stress that persists over a longer period of time ranging anywhere from two weeks to several years.

Collective personality The consistent attitude, actions, and personality traits of the people in a region.

Congruent Individual A person whose true feelings, words, and actions are all in accord.

Coping Strategies Activities taken part in for the sake of reducing the stress one incurs during the day.

Cortisol A key hormone of the stress response that is produced and released from the adrenal glands. It has many functions within the body including energy release, metabolism, acting as an anti-inflammatory, and raising blood pressure.

Conscious/Thinking Mind The part of the mind that is able to think, create, imagine, and conceive. This extension of the mind is especially pronounced in human beings, although it has been observed and proposed that a few mammals including dolphins, crows, and whales also have many conscious/thinking capabilities.

Culture The morals, values, arts, and accepted ways of being of the people in a particular area.

Delegating Passing on one's responsibilities to others, so that a balance of work between individuals can be achieved. Also called out-sourcing.

Depression A mood disorder characterized by sadness and loss of interest.

Digital Revolution The most recent revolution of human social life following both the agricultural and industrial revolution(s) of the 1900's. The digital revolution marks a shift from mechanical technology to digital electronics such as computers and cellular phones. This revolution continues through today.

Distress Negative stress. Occurs when a situation or circumstance is experienced to be outside of one's coping abilities.

Distress Load The total amount of stress that one feels.

Environmental Stress The stress which is placed on any body due to the environment around it. The weather, climate, and pollution are clear examples of environmental stress.

Eustress Positive Stress. Pushes the body into a state of excitement and the mind into a state of engagement, and is normally perceived as being enjoyed by the individual.

Existential Friction An uncomfortable feeling that the way we are living isn't in accordance with our passions, longings, and calling.

Flow A state of optimal experience characterized by the merging of task and awareness.

Food Journaling Recording what one eats for the sake of reference. If how one feels both emotionally and physically is also noticed and recorded, then insight into food choices that work well for the individual can be gathered.

Goals Unique accomplishments that people aim to either acquire or achieve, usually within a given duration of time.

Happy Hormones Hormones such as serotonin and dopamine that elevate one's mood and lead to feelings of happiness or jubilation.

Heartfelt Desires Things we wish to attain or experience that arise within the mind from an authentic intention to grow and evolve.

Higher Power Something greater than ourselves which has profound love, intelligence, and creativity.

Holistic Applies the philosophy of holism, which is that the whole of an organism or environment is greater than the sum of it's parts. Holistic actions take the health of an entire living system into account.

Holistic Society A society where the health of the people and the environment is considered pertinent in all system design.

Homeostasis A state of steady internal, physical, and chemical conditions maintained by living organisms.

Immunity The capacity of an organism to resist and neutralize infectious bacteria, viruses, and other microorganisms.

Immune System The organ system composed of the bone marrow, thyroid, lymph nodes, and kidneys that is needed for healing, repair, and defense of the body.

Inner Child A person's supposed original or true self, especially when regarded as damaged or concealed by negative childhood experiences.

Melatonin A hormone predominantly produced by the pineal gland that plays a key role in the sleep-wake cycle by aiding a person to fall asleep.

Mental/Emotional Stress The wear and tear on a physical body caused by the repetitive thinking of thoughts that cause the body to go into a state of high alert and run on 'overdrive.'

Mihaly Csikszentmihalyi Flow researcher and author who has done much of his research and work through the University of Chicago.

Mindset Shifts Changes in one's thinking that normally lead to a healthier life and improved way of viewing one's life or the world.

Minimalism An attitude of living with as few possessions as possible while still living healthily.

Money Mindset One's attitudes, beliefs, and expectations related to the concept of money.

Oxytocin A hormone released during times of bonding that creates feelings of closeness and affection. Nicknamed "the love hormone" by biologists.

People Pleasing Going to great lengths to gain the love and respect of others, even at the expense of individual needs.

Perfectionism An attitude of trying to achieve or maintain an almost impossible standard of quality in almost all areas of life.

Personality Any individuals unique behaviors, cognitions, and modes of expression.

Present-Moment-Enjoyers A nickname for people who demonstrate Type B personality qualities. The attitude of present moment enjoyment has the tendency of being stress resistant.

Relaxation Response A physical state where the parasympathetic nervous system is activated and leads to slower heart rate, slower breathing, and diversion of the blood to the internal organs. This state is usually conducive to healing and repair within the body.

Relaxation Technique Any activity we routinely take part in that triggers the relaxation response of the body.

Resilience The process of adapting well in the face of adversity, tragedy, threat, or significant sources of stress. Basically, the ability to handle and move past challenging experiences.

Schumann Resonance The natural electromagnetic frequency emitted by most natural environments.

Self-Care Actions or attitudes that people take in order to tend to their needs for health and well-being.

Sense of Self Derived from the unique person you view yourself to be with your views, values, qualities, and attributes.

Serotonin A neurotransmitter whose balanced levels help to reduce depression and anxiety and boost positive moods.

Sleep Hygiene The actions one takes which either help or hinder the quality and quantity of sleep one experiences.

Sleeping Routine The routine of when a person goes to bed, falls asleep, and rises in the morning.

Soul The eternal, timeless, and infinite part of oneself that survives physical death.

Stress Any action, event, or circumstance that throws the body, mind, or emotions out of a state of balance.
The more classic definition of stress is, "The nonspecific response of the body to any demand for change."

Stressors Actions, events, or circumstances which cause stress. These are normally 'negative' forms of stress.

Strivers Slang for people who pursue their goals with the attitude of a Type A personality. This can be a desirable quality unless striving becomes excessive.

Sub-Conscious Brain The part of the brain in charge of maintaining the body's homeostasis and responding to external stimuli. The sub-conscious brain is always attempting to maintain balance for the body, but will respond to threats by triggering the 'fight or flight' mode.

The Stress Response The response of the mind and body of an organism to either a perceived or real threat. This is normally accompanied by an increase in heart rate, blood pressure, breath rate, and a diversion of the blood and energy of the body to the arm and leg muscles.

Stress Management Routine The actions one takes on a regular basis to reduce, eliminate or better manage stress levels.

Talk Therapy A form of psychological and emotional healing that can bring relief to one who openly communicates their struggles, challenges, and difficulties.

Trauma An intensely stressful experience that leaves a long-lasting impression in the mind of the traumatized person. These experiences could be physical, mental or emotional in nature.

Trauma Recall An experience where the feelings and emotions associated with a traumatic experience are brought into present-moment awareness.

Yoga Derived from the Sanskrit terminology "to yoke together." A combination of philosophy, breathing exercises, and stretches that intend to enhance the unity between body, mind, and spirit.

Resources

Introduction

American Psychological Association, 2012. The Impact of Stress: Is Stressed Out The New Norm?. Available at: http:// stressinamerica.com [Accessed 18 July 2020].

American Psychological Association, 2017. Stress in America: 2017 Snapshot.

American Psychological Association, 2010. Stress in America Findings.

Cohen, S. and Janicki-Deverts, D., 2012. Who's Stressed? Distributions of psychological stress in the United States in probability samples from 1983, 2006 and 2009. *Journal of Applied Social Psychology*, 42(6).

Dasgupta, A., 2018. The Science Of Stress Management. Lanham: Rowman & Littlefield.

Nerurkar, A., Bitton, A., Davis, R., Phillips, R. and Yeh, G., 2013. When Physicians Counsel About Stress: Results of a National Study. *JAMA Internal Medicine*, 173(1), p.76.

Taris, T., 2016. Work & Stress: Thirty years of impact. *Work & Stress*, 30(1), pp.1-6.

Part 1

Allen, R. J. (1983). Human stress: Its nature and control. Minneapolis, MN: Burgess.

Alter, B., & Alter, S. (2019, March 1). 5 Lifestyle Tips To Nourish Your Adrenals. Retrieved August 23, 2020, from https:// www.alter.health/blog/5-lifestyle-tips-to-nourish-your-adrenals

Betts, J. G., Wise, J., Young, K. A., Desaix, P., Johnson, E., Johnson, J. E., . . . Betts, J. G. (2017). *Anatomy and physiology*. Acton, MA: XanEdu.

Brown, Selkurt, E., 1984. *Physiology*. Boston: Little, Brown.L

Csikszentmihalyi, M. (2009). Flow: The psychology of optimal experience. New York: Harper Row.

Dacher, E. S. (1993). PNI: The new mind/body healing program. New York, NY: Paragon House.

Gass, G. H., & Kaplan, H. M. (1996). *Handbook of endocrinology.* Boca Raton: CRC Press.

Jenkins, G. (2016). Anatomy and physiology. Hoboken: John Wiley.

Joubert, D. F. (2011). Tend and befriend: A bio-behavioural construction of womens responses to stress.

Lazarus, R. S. (2006). Stress and emotion: A new synthesis. New York (N.Y.): Springer.

Levine, P. A., & Maté, G. (2010). In an unspoken voice how the body releases trauma and restores goodness. Berkeley, CA: North Atlantic Books.

Matthews, J., Bryant, C., Skinner, J., & Green, D. (2019). *The Professional's Guide to Health and Wellness Coaching.* San Diego, CA: ACE.

Maté, G. (2019). When the body says no: The cost of hidden stress. Brunswick, Victoria, Australia: Scribe.

Rushkoff, D. (2013). Present Shock: When Everything Happens Now. New York: Current.

Scott, E. (2019, October 08). How to Reduce the Effects of Stress on Your Life. Retrieved from https://www.verywellmind.com/stress-management-4157211

Seaward, B., 2015. *Managing Stress.* 8th ed. Burlington: Jones & Bartlett Learning.

Selye, H. (1984). *The stress of life.* New York: The McGraw-Hill.

Taylor, S. E. (2002). Tending Instinct: Women, Men and the Biology of Nurturing. New York: Times Books.

Tintera, J. (1955). The Hypoadrenia Cortical State and its Management. *New York State Journal of Medicine, 55*(13).

Tolle, E. (2004). *The power of now: A guide to spiritual enlightenment.* Berkeley, Calif: Distributed to the trade by Group West.

Wilson, J. L. (2017). Adrenal fatigue: The 21st century stress syndrome. Petaluma, CA: Smart Publications.

Part 2

Albom, Mitch. Tuesdays with Morrie an Old Man, a Young Man, and Lifes Greatest Lesson. Sphere, 2017.

Ben-Shahar, Tal. The Pursuit of Perfect: How to Stop Chasing Perfection and Start Living a Richer, Happier Life. McGraw-Hill, 2009.

Dasgupta, A., 2018. The Science Of Stress Management. Lanham: Rowman & Littlefield.

Frankl, V. E. (2000). Mans search for meaning: An introduction to logotherapy. New York: Houghton, Mifflin.

Hiresuccess. "Understanding the 4 Personality Types: A, B, C, and D: Hire Success®." *Understanding the 4 Personality Types: A, B, C, and D | Hire Success®*, www.hiresuccess.com/help/understanding-the-4-personality-types.

Matthews, J., Bryant, C., Skinner, J., & Green, D. (2019). *The Professional's Guide to Health and Wellness Coaching*. San Diego, CA: ACE.

Schultz, Duane P., and Sydney Ellen Schultz. *Theories of Personality*. Cengage Learning, 2017.

Seligman, Martin E. P. *Authentic Happiness*. Random House Australia, 2011.

Stress and Osteoporosis. (2017, July 25). Retrieved from https://www.oamichigan.com/stress-and-osteoporosis/

Tannis, A. (2013, April 28). What Is Adrenal Fatigue? Retrieved from https://www.youtube.com/watch?v=ldyrFOe0n3U

Yogi, M. (1995). The Science of Being and Art of Living. New York: Penguin Group.

Part 3

Bellet, Samuel, et al. "Effect of Physical Exercise on Adrenocortical Excretion." *Metabolism*, vol. 18, no. 6, 1969, pp. 484–487.

Benson, Herbert, and Miriam Z. Klipper. *The Relaxation Response.* Harper, 2001.

Berger, B. "Stress Reduction Through Exercise." *Motor Skills: Theory Into Pracice*, vol. 7, no. 2, 1983.

Bliss, E. (1980). Getting Things Done: The ABC's of Time Management. New York: Bantam Books.

Boyes, Carolyn. Cognitive Behavioural Therapy. Collins, 2008.

Buzzell, Linda. Ecotherapy: Healing with Nature in Mind. Sierra Club Books, 2009.

Cameron, Julia. Artists Way: 25th Anniversary Edition. Penguin Books, 2016.

Campbell, D. *The Mozart Effect.* Avon Books, 1997.

Campbell, Joseph. The Hero with a Thousand Faces. Yogi Impressions, 2017.

Cohen, Kenneth S. *The Way of Qigong.* Random House International, 2000.

Cooper, Kenneth H. *The New Aerobics.* Evans, New York. 1970

Covey, S. R. (2020). The 7 habits of highly effective people: Powerful lessons in personal change. New York: Simon & Schuster.

Dacher, E. S. (1993). PNI: The new mind/body healing program. New York, NY: Paragon House.

Duhigg, Charles. *The Power Of Habit.* Random House, 2014.

Floyd, J, et al. "The Effect of Music, Imagery, and Relaxation on Adrenal Corticostreroids and the Re-Entrainment of Circadian Rhythms." *The Journal of Music Therapy*, vol. 22, 1985.

Fogg, Brian J. Tiny Habits: the Small Changes That Change Everything. Virgin Books, 2019.

Publishing, H. H. (2020, July 7). Exercising to Relax. Retrieved from https://www.health.harvard.edu

Hạnh Nhất, and Lilian W. Y. Cheung. *Savor: Mindful Eating, Mindful Life*. HarperOne, 2011.

Hill, N. *Think and grow rich*. (1966). New York: Hawthorn Books.

Ilardi, S. S. (2019). The depression cure: The six-step programme to beat depression without drugs. London: Vermilion.

Lamb, David R. Physiology of Exercise: Responses & Adaptations. Macmillan, 1984. "Joseph Campbell and the Power of Myth." PBS, 1988. Video.

Lazarus, Richard S., and Susan Folkman. *Stress, Appraisal, and Coping*. Springer, 1984.

Lazarus, Richard S. "The Stress and Coping Paradigm." *Models for Clinical Psychopathology*, 1981, pp. 177–214.

Martin, Garry, and Joseph Pear. Behavior Modification: What It Is and How to Do It. Routledge, 2019.

Matthews, J., Bryant, C., Skinner, J., & Green, D. (2019). *The Professional's Guide to Health and Wellness Coaching*. San Diego, CA: ACE.

McKay, Matthew, et al. *Messages: the Communications Skills Book*. New Harbinger Publications, Inc., 2018.

Monroe, S. IAWP Wellness Coach Training Program.

Morgan, W.P. "Exercise as a Relaxation Technique." *Primary Cardiology*, vol. 6, 1980.

Osho. (2001). Intimacy: Trusting oneself and the other: Insights for a new way of living. New York: St. Martins Griffin.

Osho. (2002). Love, freedom, aloneness: The Koan of relationships. New York: St. Martins Griffin.

Physical Activity Guidelines for Americans. 2nd ed. Available at health.gov.

Ramsey, D. (2015). Dave Ramseys complete guide to money: The handbook of Financial Peace University. Brentwood, TN: Ramsey Press.

"Robert Peng's QiGong Ecstasy." 2006. DVD.

Robinson, L., Segal, R., & Smith, M. (n.d.). How to Sleep Better. Retrieved from https://www.helpguide.org

Rockwood, L. TEDx: Change Your Breath, Change Your Life.TEDxTalks. YouTube, 10 Dec. 2018, www.youtube.com.

Rosenberg, M. B., & Gandhi, A. (2015). Non-violent communication: A language of life. Encinitas, CA: PuddleDancer Press.

Seaward, B., 2015. *Managing Stress*. 8th ed. Burlington: Jones & Bartlett Learning.

Suni, E. How Much Sleep Do We Really Need? (2020, October 09). Retrieved from https://www.sleepfoundation.org/articles/how-much-sleep-do-we-really-need

Springer, Verlag, 2011. The Power of Human Imagination New Methods in Psychotherapy.

Svoboda, R., & Svoboda, R. (2005). Prakriti: Your ayurvedic constitution. Delhi: Motilal Banarsidass.

Swanson, John L. Communing with Nature: a Guidebook for Enhancing Your Relationship with the Living Earth. Illahee Press, 2001.

Taylor, S. E. (2002). Tending Instinct: Women, Men and the Biology of Nurturing. New York: Times Books.

Twist, L., & Barker, T. (2003). The soul of money: Transforming your relationship with money and life. New York: Norton.

Uvnäs Moberg K, Handlin L, Kendall-Tackett K, Petersson M. Oxytocin is a principal hormone that exerts part of its effects by active fragments. Med Hypotheses. (2019 Dec.)

Uvnas-Moberg, K., & Petersson, M. (2018). Oxytocin, a mediator of anti-stress, well-being, social interaction, growth and healing.

Weil, Andrew. *Spontaneous Healing*. Random House, 1995.

Yogani. Deep Meditation: Pathway to Personal Freedom. AYP Publishing, 2005.

Part 4

Rollnick, S., Miller, W. R., & Butler, C. C. (2008). Motivational interviewing in health care: Helping patients change behavior. New York: Guilford.

Monroe, S. (2020) IAWP Wellness Coach Training Program.

www.ingramcontent.com/pod-product-compliance
Lightning Source LLC
Chambersburg PA
CBHW061338250726
48657CB00004B/1220